THE MICROBE FACTOR

Enzymes that Switch on Your Innate Immunity

Hiromi Shinya, MD

MILLICHAP BOOKS

Millichap Books, LLC
www.millichapbooks.com
www.enzymefactor.com

Printed in the USA

Cover and interior design by Carl Brune

ISBN 978-0-9822900-4-0 (paperback)

ISBN 978-0-9822900-6-4 (ebook)

Library of Congress Cataloging-in-Publication Data
Shinya, Hiromi.
The microbe factor your innate immunity and the coming health
revolution / Hiromi Shinya. -- 1st ed.
    p. cm.
ISBN 978-0-9822900-0-2 (hardcover : alk. paper)
1. Intestines--Microbiology. 2. Digestive enzymes. 3. Health.
4. Natural immunity. I. Title.
QR171.I6S55 2010
612.3'3--dc22

                          2010009990

Notice: This book is intended as a reference volume only, not as a medical manual. The information presented here is designed to help you make informed decisions about your health. It is not intended as a substitute for any treatment that may have been prescribed by your doctor, who is acquainted with your specific needs. If you suspect that you have a medical problem, we urge you to seek competent medical care.

Contents

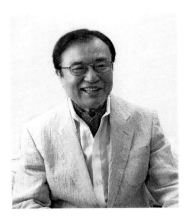

Hiromi Shinya, MD, is one of the world's leading gastroenterologists. His book *The Enzyme Factor* has sold millions of copies in the United States, Japan, and other countries. In the early 1960s Dr. Shinya pioneered the "Shinya Technique," the now-standard procedure for the removal of polyps from the colon without invasive surgery. Over a career of 40 years Dr. Shinya has treated thousands of patients. It has been his routine to get diet and nutrition histories from his patients and, by comparing this with the evidence of their colonoscopies, he has developed a set of lifestyle and diet suggestions that will enable us to live a vital, healthy life into a good old age. He has named this lifestyle the "Shinya Biozyme."

Dr. Shinya is retired as Chief of the Surgical Endoscopy Unit at New York's Beth Israel Medical Center, and Clinical Professor of Surgery at the Albert Einstein College of Medicine also in New York. Until his recent retirement, he worked with patients daily, practicing medicine in the United States and Japan.

Introduction

THE COMING HEALTH REVOLUTION

There is a health care revolution coming to the United States and the rest of the world.

I am not talking about the debates that have gone on for the past few years about national health insurance, or who pays for your prescription drugs. The health care revolution that is just now beginning will be much less about who pays for your care if you get sick and much *more* about keeping you off drugs and out of hospitals.

In my opinion as a physician in practice for almost 50 years in the United States, our current approach to health care, with its expensive array of technology and pharmaceuticals, is due for a complete overhaul — and the sooner the better. It is time we started basing our health care discussions around health, rather than illness. How can we all enjoy a full span of years with vitality?

This book is my prescription for just such ageless living. Based on the very latest (and some of the most ancient) knowledge about our bodies and how they work, I am suggesting what I call the "Shinya Biozyme," a new way of eating and living that can make you healthy and keep you healthy with a minimum of pharmaceutical and surgical interference.

We are now beginning to realize the ultimate futility of a continued war on microbes, and the focus is changing to how to maximize the "good" bacteria always present in the human body. You may have heard about the Asian concept of "chi" or "ki," a life force that flows throughout all living beings. I'll show you what this energy force really is, and how to bring "plant power" into your cellular "power plant," to maximize the life force inside the cells of your body. Speaking of life on the cellular level, I will explain how cells clean and rejuvenate themselves. You'll get a clear explanation of the latest biological research and what it tells us about the body's natural systems for rejuvenation. You'll learn how to have young cells, even into "old age."

The coming health revolution will begin with the new knowledge we have about our bodies and a new attitude emerging in the world today. Despite our technologies and the virtual-reality world in which we live, we are not separate from our environment, nor can we talk about "ecology" without reference to ourselves and our bodies. Based on the latest research – discoveries for which Nobel Prizes have recently been awarded – and based on my own clinical research over the past five decades, I have compiled a set of suggestions for eating and living that will go a long way toward keeping you youthful, vital, with a minimum of disease. I cover many issues in this book but they are not difficult to grasp, if you come with an open mind. The information that follows should be approached in the same way I advise you to approach your daily food: take it in slowly and chew it thoroughly for digestion and absorption. My hope is that you will read this book in this way, and, having read it, you will put my Biozyme prescription into practice. It is my intention that my words might nourish your mind, even as good food and good water nourish your body.

No matter your current age, living conditions, health insurance coverage, or state of health, you will find something in this book you can put into practice to improve your energy and health. Put the *entire* Shinya Biozyme into practice, make it your way of life, and you may well need no expensive pharmaceuticals or surgeries to sustain your life and health in the coming years.

Part One

THE SCIENCE OF NATURAL IMMUNITY

Chapter 1

A New View of the Human Body

A new paradigm for human health must begin with a new view of human beings and our place in the natural world. Here in the United States many people talk about their concern for the environment; books are written about ecological balance and the consequences to the planet of global climate change. Not as widely recognized is the fact that our bodies are also an ecological system and are very much a part of the earth on which we live.

As I witness the ongoing debate about health care in the United States I see that one key to this discussion is missing. Before we can see our way clear to better health care, I believe it is important to understand and to feel our individual connection to the larger whole — especially through our intestines. Okay, so I'm a gastroenterologist and maybe my viewpoint is skewed by my half century of practicing medicine specializing in the human digestive system. Still, I know that our intestines are not just long, narrow tubes. They are our primary connecting point to the earth.

Our world is alive because of microorganisms, the original life forms found everywhere from deep-sea vents to polar icecaps. These organisms collectively form an interconnected layer of life on every surface of our planet. In turn, our intestines connect us with microorganisms. Most readers already know that intestinal bacteria, both good bacteria and bad bacteria, are key to health, but my focus is not limited to that internal universe. The universe I am talking about is much vaster. The soil in which vegetables we eat grow is abuzz with the activities of microorganisms. The quality of this soil environment has a direct impact upon the quality of the food it produces, and our consumption of this food determines the condition of our intestines and ultimately of our health.

Every day the food we eat must be converted into energy. The intestines perform this vital task where the foods we eat are digested and absorbed by the blood vessels that connect the intestines to the cells in the entire body. The collective body of these forty to sixty trillion cells makes up a human — a living being.

The intestines are also the place in the body where enzymes are created. These enzymes are the impetus for every action inside our cells. To be full of the energy of life means that the cells of the entire body are active and are providing energy. You've heard it many times before: You are what you eat. Perhaps this statement has been repeated so often it no longer has the power to capture your attention, but it is no less true. What (and how) you eat impacts both your body and your mind.

In the practice of modern medicine, prescriptions and surgery are the leading treatments. It is rare to have a doctor recommend a dietary health management program focusing on the way we absorb the life energy in food into the body, and aimed at improving the health of intestines. Instead, physicians and patients alike seem preoccupied with eliminating immediate symptoms without an understanding of the real causes of disease. With its expensive medicines and technologies the American system has created a health-care model that only the wealthy can afford, but even at these high prices is our system really caring for our health?

I believe health care should start with the digestive system and the food we put into it. In this book I will show how the intestines are our vital connection to the energy of the universe and how we can build and maintain our health by strengthening this connection.

My earlier book, *The Enzyme Factor,* published both in Japan and in the United States, has sparked an increasing interest in these dietary and health recommendations. Because of it many people have incorporated these recommendations into their daily lives.

Over my half century in the practice of medicine, I have taken the dietary histories of thousands of people while comparing their diets to the features of their intestines. This has given me a great understanding of the relationship between diet, intestinal health, and the health of the rest of the body. I have been convinced by a mountain of clinical evidence that the view through my endoscopic instrument, whether the intestines I see are clean or dirty, healthy or unhealthy, will depend upon what the patient habitually eats. The condition of the intestines, in turn, will determine the condition of the blood that carries vital nutrients to every cell of the body. I believe you can live a long and healthy life with no serious illness … but only if you have the "guts" of a healthy eater.

The Shinya health method, which I call the Shinya Biozyme, is packed with secrets for achieving healthy intestines, healthy blood and vibrant cells. Speaking from the point of view of the intestines you will learn why some widely accepted nutritional advice is actually harmful to many people. More importantly, you'll learn what is good to eat and why. You'll also learn how to listen and respond to your own body and become aware of the language of your gut in order to drastically improve your health.

Much of my research has focused on the enzymes that are working inside cells. I have tried to conceptualize them by calling them "newzymes" because they are the enzymes that are constantly at work renewing the body. Newzymes are at the root of our life force and vitality. If you examine the activities of cells with newzymes as the focus, you will come to realize why so many of us have lost energy and have regressed in motivation and creative vitality. You will understand the problems caused by trying to replace this natural life force with stimulants like caffeine, sugar, and even more unhealthy substances.

Our national obsession with physical appearance and "beauty" is yet another way in which we are waging war against nature. We use everything from fat burners to implants to botox in order to look younger and more attractive than we naturally are. Yet, in the true sense, beauty is the same thing as natural health. Throughout the animal kingdom, beauty is the outward sign of health and vitality. Furry animals are most attracted to mates whose fur is shiny and eyes are clear and bright. It is nature's way of promoting the propagation of the healthiest of each species.

Making peace with nature, then, means a new "beauty" regime based on healthy eating and living. A healthy lifestyle will improve not only your "inner face" — your intestinal tract, but will make your outer face more beautiful as well. A healthy inner face is also reflected as a natural richness of heart, a sense of security, and the strength of self-confidence.

Of course, if you go on an extreme diet, giving no thought to the health of your intestines, you may succeed at weight loss. If you lose five pounds in a month, you may feel a sense of accomplishment and this may boost your confidence. However, unless such a diet method includes a change to a healthy lifestyle, you cannot achieve any kind of real beauty. If you have gained confidence from such an achievement, it will be temporary. After a while, the weight lost will rebound making it necessary to jump at a new diet method. The reason the effects of most diet methods are temporary is because they fail to improve the intestines, which are the foundation of the health of both body and mind. If you want to be a really beautiful woman or attractive man, you must pay attention to your intestines before anything else.

Men and women with so called "potbellies" are likely suffering from metabolic syndrome, also called insulin resistance syndrome, a combination of medical disorders that increase the risk of developing cardiovascular disease and diabetes. It affects one in five people, and prevalence increases with age. Some studies estimate the prevalence in the USA to be as high as 25% of the population. Recent research indicates that prolonged stress can be an underlying cause of metabolic syndrome by upsetting the hormonal balance of the Hypothalamic-pituitary-adrenal axis (HPA-axis). Such an effort as limiting calorie intake or strenuous, unfamiliar exercise will put unnatural stress on the body. Behind the issue of weight or body fat is the problem of one's lifestyle. In other words, an unnatural diet has stressed the body and brought about the deterioration of intestinal features, which in turn has caused obesity, aging of the skin and many other unhealthy conditions of the body.

Our lifestyle and our approach to health care has become divorced from nature, and has relied on our ability to use science and technology *against* nature — our own physical nature and the natural world in which we live. Today we can use science and technology to cooperate with nature. We, ourselves, are part of the natural world, and real health care in the future will have to begin with a recognition and full acceptance of that fact.

As long as we continue to speak and think of health as a war on nature, we will be fighting against our own flesh and "fouling the nest" in which we live. In the long run, we will be the losers. Nowhere is this clearer than in relation to our battle against pathogens. It is time to make friends with the microbes that live all around us and inside us.

Chapter 2

The War on Microbes

For the past hundred years or so, the medical and health care establishment has been in a state of war against nature.

When I began my practice of surgery and gastroenterology in New York back in the mid-1960s, the feeling was that we were winning that war. With antibiotics we had conquered a whole host of infectious diseases that had plagued humans down through the ages. Vaccinations had made smallpox, tetanus, diphtheria, polio, and other dread infections a thing of the past. Better surgical techniques were allowing doctors to reach into the body and repair or remove diseased organs – and even replace them with transplants and artificial spare parts.

The "miracle of modern medicine" seemed on the verge of wiping out diseases of every kind and the average life expectancy for my generation soared. One crucial aspect of this "miracle" was the widespread acceptance of the germ model of disease. Microbes, popularly called germs, were held responsible for most diseases. Kill off the germs, or harness the body's own army of antibodies to kill them, and we could live free of disease. We also learned to halt dread diseases like malaria and bubonic plague by killing the insects and vermin that spread them.

The medical establishment was winning in the life-and-death struggle by means of scientific search-and-destroy tactics. Researchers would search out the microbial causes of disease and develop weapons to destroy them. Then doctors and public health workers would use these weapons to kill the "bad germs" in their patients, enabling the sick to recover and the healthy to stay well.

The result of humankind's war on microbes was so spectacularly successful that we could begin to turn our attention to the conquest of all disease. We declared "war" on cancer, heart disease, and lung disease.

But then we found that there were no microbial enemies we could search out to destroy in order to cure these diseases. Instead, we have discovered that many of our deadliest ailments are related to poor diet, lack of exercise, smoking, drinking and other lifestyle issues. The battleground in the war against disease has shifted. In the words of Walt Kelly's comic-strip character, Pogo, "We have met the enemy and he is us."

Meanwhile, some of the microbes we thought we'd conquered began to make a comeback. We began to see more new types of influenza for which we had no vaccine. We began to see drug-resistant forms of pneumonia, tuberculosis, and other infectious diseases. It began to dawn on everybody that microbes, like every other life form, have the ability to evolve and adapt. We can keep developing new drugs to fight them, but we will only hasten the evolution of super-bugs for which there may be no cure. Perhaps it is time for all of us to stop thinking in terms of medical warfare and take a different approach to human health.

One approach might be to get rid of the warfare model altogether. This mindset has taken us a long way in our quest for health, but it stems from an incomplete picture of how our bodies work.

MICROORGANISMS WITH THE POWER OF LIFE AND DEATH

All of us who are born into the world are controlled by living organisms that cannot be seen with our human eyes. These organisms hold power over our life. I am talking about microorganisms, so small they can be seen only with the eyes of science. Microorganisms inhabit our bodies at all times; in fact they inhabit all places on the earth. Microorganisms exist outside our bodies and they exist inside our bodies.

Some microorganisms cannot exist independently and must propagate in the cells of other organisms, and others can live independently as organisms.

Of the first group, virus, rickettsia, and chlamydia are examples. These microorganisms have the characteristic of being parasitic on other organisms to propagate. There are arguments as to whether this group may even be classified as organisms; they look sort of like organisms and sort of not. A virus, for example, does not have a cell, often thought of as the most basic unit of life.

The second category of microorganisms, composed of cells, can live independently. There are two types of cells. Prokaryotes do not have cell nuclei, while eukaryotic cells do. Bacteria are a large group of unicellular prokaryote microorganisms. All complex multicellular organisms, including fungi, plants, animals, and humans, are composed of eukaryotic cells. Everything alive that we can see, from the tall trees to a beloved pet to ourselves in the mirror, is made from the same kind of complex cell. Microorganisms, on the other hand, may or may not be.

Although they are extremely small and are barely visible through a microscope, microorganisms have the strength of numbers. Presently the explosion of human population is an issue, but human population is nothing compared to the populations of microorganisms on earth. There are 100 million to 1 billion microbes in a single gram of fertile soil, and 100 trillion of them in the intestines of a human being.

Of course we don't see this vast population because they are almost infinitesimally small. A bacterium is 1 over 500–2000 millimeters, a yeast of the fungi family measures 1 over 5,000 millimeters, and a virus measures 1 over several tens of thousands to several hundreds of thousands millimeters.

The existence of such a vast number of microorganisms implies that they have an excellent capacity to adapt to changes in their environment. With regard to temperature, for example, these microorganisms are broadly classified into the groups of cryophiles which propagate at temperatures below 77° F, mesophiles which propagate at 77 to 100° F, and thermophiles, which propagate at between 113 and 176 °F.

Microorganisms that can propagate at high temperatures exceeding 194 °F were discovered recently. Also there are salt-loving organisms, which thrive where saline concentration is high, sweet-loving organisms, which thrive in high concentrations of glucose, acidophiles which favor acidic environments with low pH, while others favor alkaline environments high in pH, anaerobes which can survive without oxygen, and aerobes which thrive in environments with good ventilation. Clearly, living organisms can survive in a wide range of environments.

We are coexisting on our planet earth with these vast numbers and types of microorganisms, all multiplying and prospering around and through us. Unless we know about them we cannot know the truth about our own world. From our point of view as human beings, there is both a bright side and a dark side to sharing the planet with microorganisms. By viewing both sides we will come to understand a little better how we can thrive on a living earth.

THE DEADLY IMPACT OF VIRUSES

It probably will come as no surprise to you that humans have been threatened throughout our existence by diseases caused by pathogen microorganisms. Viruses are the typical example.

Viruses are neither organic nor inorganic. They neither metabolize nor breathe by themselves, and they are parasitic in the cells of other organisms, propagating inside the cells of the host. In the process, they destroy these cells and the newly propagated viruses move on to invade new cells and propagate again. As the result of such propagation, the host will develop various diseases, such as the flu or the common cold. Sometimes the host dies, but even this death will not stop the viruses from jumping to a new, healthy host to propagate again. Contagious diseases brought on by viruses have rampaged throughout all parts of the world since ancient times.

The virus that causes influenza triggers severe symptoms, while a cold generally affects the nose and throat. The influenza virus has a short incubation stage of about a week after initial infection then symptoms such as fever, fatigue, and joint pains appear. Most of the time flu doesn't kill, but it can be an extremely serious disease nonetheless, causing complications like bronchitis and pneumonia, triggering encephalitis.

The Spanish flu which spread throughout the world in 1918-1920 is well known. In those days, nobody knew that it was caused by a virus. A staggering 30% of the world population was infected. In the United States 500,000-675,000 died; worldwide, the death toll is estimated at 50 million to 100 million. More recently, we have been hit with other virus-related diseases. Aside from influenza, there were AIDS (acquired immune deficiency syndrome), which destroys all the immune functions of the body, SARS (severe acute respiratory syndrome), which rampaged in China, Hong Kong and Taiwan, and norovirus which affected 10 million people or more in 2006. Among influenza, in 2004, infection of Bird Flu was confirmed in Japan for the first time in 80 years and poultry producers had to dispose of large quantity of infected birds. In 2009 and 2010 the H1N1 virus (Swine Flu) spread around the globe. Smallpox and measles are viral contagious diseases. They are now considered to be almost extinct, but they used to be a threat to many.

The challenging aspect of most virus-related diseases is that we have little knowledge of such vital information as their cycle, timing, and the transmission routes of respective epidemics. Furthermore, we have not really found decisive measures to deal with virus-related diseases or their spread. Preventive vaccinations are recommended against influenza, but, as the flu virus is so quick to mutate, they are far from an absolute solution.

MICROORGANISMS AND HUMAN HISTORY

Microorganisms called pathogens are not limited to viruses. Tuberculosis, cholera, plague, dysentery, syphilis, and tetanus are all infections caused by microorganisms. Also, rickettsia and chlamydia are known as pathogens causing infectious diseases.

These contagious diseases have had a profound impact on human history. The plague known as the Black Death swept throughout Europe in the middle of the fourteenth century. We now know that fleas bearing plague bacillus caused its spread. One third of the 100 million Europeans or 30 million people lost their lives in the Black Death plague.

The symptoms of infection with a deadly virus vary. Bubonic plague causes a high fever and swelling of lymphatic glands, plague septicemia causes black spots (hemorrhagic lesions), lung plague causes pneumonia and so forth. It is assumed that the epidemic is repeated in a cycle of several hundred years. In the middle of nineteenth century Bubonic plague caused the death of approximately 12 million people in China and India.

You may think that this is a disease of the past, but it has not been eradicated completely as evidenced by the death of 50 people in India in 1994. In fact, there are quite a number of countries in Africa and South America which have been designated as plague polluted regions by WHO (World Health Organization).

Typhus fever caused by the pathogen rickettsia is known to have caused several epidemics in history. Napoleon who had taken Europe by storm was compelled to retreat not just because of the harsh winter cold, but also because of the spread of typhus fever among his men.

Smallpox and other infectious diseases caused epidemics that ravaged the Americas following first contact with Europeans. Recently anthropologists have come to believe that as much as 85 to 90 percent of the native population of the Americas was killed off by microorganisms brought by Europeans, the single most important factor in the conquest of the indigenous civilizations. Americans speak Spanish, English, Portuguese and French today because of microbes.

There are countless such cases in which contagious diseases have changed history. The smallpox vaccination method developed by a British physician, Edward Jenner, became popular all over the world, and as the result, the population of affected people declined gradually, and there was hardly anyone suffering from it by the end of World War II. The last diagnosed case of smallpox was in Somalia in 1977. This is why it is said that smallpox is the only contagious disease that humans have succeeded in eradicating.

Measles, a contagious disease caused by the measles virus, was once a common childhood ailment. Those infants and children who survived the disease developed immunity, and they did not contract the disease for the rest of their lives. Some adults who had not contracted measles in their infancy ended up dying in measles epidemics, which repeatedly swept the world.

COULD ANTIBIOTICS ERADICATE PATHOGENS?

Vaccinations can help prevent measles, but there is as yet no cure. The death rate has decreased drastically, but recently the number of adults affected by the disease has been on the rise. In 2007 an epidemic of measles hit high schools and colleges throughout Japan and more than 100 schools were compelled to close.

Why were so many young adults stricken with measles as a group? At the time, it was explained that those people infected had not received measles vaccinations in their childhood. A more thorough investigation revealed, however, that some who had received the vaccination were also the victims.

In measles vaccinations, weakened measles viruses are injected so that antibodies are created making it difficult to contract the disease. This method provides quasi-immunity and is inferior to the immunity (resistance) developed by the person who contracts the disease and overcomes it.

In the U.S. and Europe the trend is to vaccinate against measles twice, i.e., when an infant is one year old and before a child is admitted to an elementary school. The U.S. introduced this double vaccination method in 1970 with the result that the incidence rate of measles has come down drastically. By doubling the number of vaccinations, the resistance level increases, making it difficult to contract measles.

Given such a result, we have to acknowledge that vaccination is effective. Yet it seems to me that an important point is being overlooked. If we viewed our natural world as a series of inter-related systems, we might find that another approach toward disease could be more sustainable and effective.

In order to understand such an approach, it would be necessary to ask, "What is the root of the life power which supports our being?" Before we try to answer that question, however, let's review how modern medicine has been dealing with infectious diseases.

The first effort the medical establishment undertook was to "specify the cause." In the middle of nineteenth century, Louis Pasteur from France and Robert Koch from Germany established the technologies to cultivate microorganisms. This led to the discovery of a series of bacilli such as tubercle bacillus, cholera bacillus, typhoid bacillus and so forth. Japanese scholars were also active in this field, and at about the same time Shibasaburo Kitasato discovered tetanus bacillus and bubonic bacillus and Yoshi Shiga discovered *Bacillus dysentericus*. If these pathogens were removed from the body, infectious diseases might be prevented. Following this idea, antibiotics were developed.

The first antibiotic was penicillin. It was developed by a British bacteriologist, Alexander Fleming, from substances in blue mold. In a way, this was an attempt to restrain a pathogenic microbe with the work of a different microbe (blue mold). With the mass-production of penicillin, the death rate from infection dropped drastically, causing a great sensation with pronouncements such as "the greatest discovery of the twentieth century," "medical revolution," and so forth. Various researches in antibiotics followed.

Many researchers hoped and believed that the development of antibiotics would lead to a complete conquest of the infectious diseases of mankind. It took about a century for humankind to begin to wake up from this dream. A new resistant bacterium came into the picture. Then, a new antibiotic to resist this bacterium was developed followed by a new resistant bacterium and so forth. This vicious cycle is still going on.

Today, the world is faced with a new question: Is the concept of conquering pathogens with antibiotics still valid? Are we not simply breeding super bacteria against which we will find no defense?

AN ALTERNATIVE APPROACH TO
CONTROLLING INFECTIOUS DISEASES

In the past few hundred years researchers have identified many pathogens. The ones identified, however, represent only a minute portion of the countless microorganisms in our world. Even when an antibiotic effective against a certain infectious disease is developed, it is only a drop in the ocean of the activities of microorganisms. Antibiotics, to be sure, are a great advancement in health care, but they are not the complete answer to contagious diseases. For one thing, we have not developed a full understanding of these microbes; in fact it would be almost impossible to gain a full understanding of the scope of their being.

We should not forget that we as human beings are a part of nature and that we live within the realm of its rules. Unless we have respect for nature and humility before its forces, any medicine we might produce would only be an ad hoc solution leading to a counterattack by nature. The endless race between resistant bacteria and antibiotics is just one example of this truth.

The treatment for tuberculosis is another. Tuberculosis has been on the rise for the past few years. This contagious killer disease is caused by tubercle bacillus. Until 1950, it was the number one cause of death in Japan. After the war brought the widespread use of antibiotics such as streptomycin, the number of tuberculosis patients dropped drastically. For a while tuberculosis was regarded as "a disease of the past." Recently, however, the population of infected persons is on the rise again, especially among the elderly and young people.

To cope with this situation, BCG (Bacillus Calmette-Guérin) vaccination is recommended in Japan, though not in the United States where there is currently a low risk of tuberculosis infection. Even this vaccination is not 100% effective. When a person is infected with tuberculosis, tubercle bacilli remain in his lung, and as the effectiveness of the vaccination diminishes and the resistance of the patient becomes weak, there have been cases in which tubercle bacilli suddenly commence propagation, causing the onset of the disease. Some attribute the recent increase of tuberculosis to the change in effectiveness of vaccination, but I wonder if this is the only answer.

The bacteria called tubercle bacilli are found in nature. Perhaps many of us have contracted tubercle bacilli without being aware of it. Contracting the bacilli does not necessarily lead to the onset of the disease. Statistically speaking it is said that 1 out of 10 persons who contracts tubercle bacilli show the symptoms, and even if one shows the symptoms, the effect could be mild. There are, however, over 2,000 deaths from tuberculosis every year.

Where is the difference among individuals contracting the tubercle bacilli? The difference is the resistance (immune strength) of individuals.

A strong immune system will reduce the chances of contracting diseases. This is not limited to tuberculosis, but applies to all contagious diseases. Inevitably, our attempts to destroy pathogens will end up in a race we will lose. The only way for us to win against disease is by strengthening the human immune system.

The increasing number of people with tuberculosis is a sign that our powers of resistance may be in decline, making us more prone to all diseases. Rather than solely relying on challenging microorganisms with antibiotics, isn't there another healthcare approach that is more in line with natural laws? Preventive medicine must surely be part of the answer to that question.

When you trace human history, you will see that our ancestors had to cope with severe environments. Life was hard; there might have been inadequate shelter from cold or heat, grinding poverty, filthy living conditions, and deprivations of every sort with any number of negative results. Even now, there are many countries where the average life span is only 30 years. In the Meiji era, in Japan, both men and women on average lived only to their late thirties. The average life span in Japan has more than doubled and Japan is now called the country with the highest level of longevity in the world, even as longevity in the United States lags behind.

What is the reason for this? Is it attributable to the economic growth from modernization? The Edo era in Japan, running from 1603 to 1868, was a time of peace and prosperity. There was no widespread poverty or starvation. The cultural life flourished and farming was popular. In some ways, it was an era more economically prosperous than today. And yet, the average life span was much shorter.

The reason is simple. The rate of infant death from such diseases as smallpox or measles was overwhelmingly high. This is certainly a miserable situation, and yet if you take another view, those who survived the infections built immunity against many diseases. In a way, those individuals who survived to adulthood were the chosen ones. They were likely much heartier, healthier and energetic than we are today. As killer diseases heartlessly weeded out the weakest among us, nature bred a disease-resistant population.

To say that the average lifespan was in the thirties does not mean that everyone died in his thirties; that was just a lifespan figure reached by averaging all the infant mortality with the lifespan of those few who made it to adulthood. There must have been a large number who lived into their seventies and eighties with more vigor than most older people today. If we are blinded by the average lifespan figures, we will fail to understand the physical strength of the average adult survivors.

We have attained many conveniences in life through rapid modernization. Because of infrastructures such as sewage systems, public hygiene has greatly improved, cutting back on infectious diseases that spread in unsanitary environments. The rampage of plague in Europe in the middle ages was partially attributable to the environment. The Europeans did not have toilets and simply dumped their waste in sewage canals beside their houses and drank from rivers were filled with filthy water. The large numbers of rodents in such an environment carried pest bacilli to various areas, quickly spreading deadly illnesses.

In addition to the establishment of public health sanitation, antibiotics and vaccinations became popular after World War II, and as a result the number of people infected by contagious diseases has drastically declined. The longevity we have achieved in this way, however, means that many who might have died in infancy or childhood were saved, despite a weaker immune system that would have made them susceptible to fatal infectious diseases, had they been exposed. Others who would have survived these diseases and built up an immunity remain vulnerable into adulthood, having never had the chance to encounter certain microbes and create the necessary antibodies.

"Gringos" who travel to countries south of the border are warned not to drink the water there because it is full of bacteria that will probably make them quite ill with "Montezuma's Revenge." The natives in these countries, however, seem to be able to drink this water and cook with it with few or no ill effects. This is because they are used to it. They have been exposed to the bacteria in the water repeatedly since infancy and developed immunity to its ill effects.

It seems our sanitary conditions and the modern medicines with which we once thought to have conquered infectious diseases have actually made us weaker, as a population, and more vulnerable to disease. Our vulnerability is an unintended consequence of the advance of medicine and our desire to free ourselves from suffering and death from disease.

Of course, there is no need for us to abandon the advantages brought by civilization and modernization. No one wants to return to the days when it was a common thing to lose children to infectious diseases. We should be thankful and enjoy the affluence we have obtained. At the same time we should perhaps relearn the ancient wisdom that the most important thing we can do for ourselves, our families and our larger group is to develop a strong, healthy body with strong immune power. Our ancestors had to conquer hunger and poverty. Our challenge is to regain the natural vigor of the human organism.

The key to accomplishing this lies in our daily lifestyle and, prosaically enough, in the heath of our intestines. We can live to a good old age with amazing health and vitality … if we have the guts.

THE GIFT OF MICROORGANISMS

Even as modern medicine wages war against the microbes that sicken and kill, we have come to understand that, by and large, microbes are our friends. In fact, without them we wouldn't be able to grow, digest and metabolize our food.

There is an inseparable relationship between our intestines and microorganisms. In explaining the activities of bacteria in the body, we often divide intestinal microorganisms into "beneficial bacteria" and "harmful bacteria." To be more accurate, however, most of our intestinal flora are intermediate bacteria, opportunistic microorganisms, which do not belong in either category.

The proportion of bacteria in our intestines is approximately 20% beneficial bacteria, 30% harmful bacteria, with the remaining 50% being intermediate bacteria. The key bacteria that contribute to the control of the intestinal environment are the *intermediate* bacteria. This is because, when the proportion of harmful bacteria increases as the result of irregular meals and other bad eating habits, intermediate bacteria are drawn into the domain of harmful bacteria and the majority of intestinal bacteria act as harmful bacteria, decomposing undigested foods and generating toxic gas. Given this bad environment, in time the intestinal features deteriorate and various diseases begin to show up.

On the other hand, when the proportion of beneficial bacteria increases, intermediate bacteria are synchronized with beneficial bacteria and, as a result, the intestines will be inhabited by countless beneficial bacteria, soon bringing about a stable intestinal environment. Over time, the intestinal features become clean, and the person is much more likely to enjoy a long and healthy life, mentally and physically.

You might think of the intermediate bacteria as the swing voters in an election.

Actually, my segregation of intestinal bacteria into "beneficial" and "harmful" is for descriptive convenience only. Remember, the majority of bacteria that inhabit human intestines are bacteria in the gray zone—intermediate bacteria—neither good nor bad. They will become either beneficial or harmful when triggered by a slight change in the environment. The real swing voter, then is *you*.

How do you support beneficial bacteria in your intestines in order to live a healthy life? Health is not a matter of destroying all harmful bacteria in your intestines, but of living and eating in a way that keeps the intermediate bacteria from "going bad." One way to do this is by eating fermented foods.

FERMENTATION

Microbes cause food to spoil, but they also can be used as preservatives, and people learned to do this very early in human history, using bacteria for fermentation. Fermented foods and drink are found in dietary cultures around the world.

Lactobacillus is a typical beneficial bacteria in human intestines. It is also the bacteria necessary for fermenting yogurt or cheese and for making Japanese miso (soy bean paste), soy sauce, pickles, and vinegar. Though all these foods are fermented using the same lactobacillus group, there is a big difference in that yogurt and cheese are derived from milk from animals, while miso paste and soy sauce are derived from plants. The lactobacillus in the vinegar used in making sauerkraut produces lactic acid, which inhibits the growth of other microorganisms. In the preparation of miso and soy sauce, not only lactobacillus but also various microorganisms such as koji and yeast bacillus are used. Among the soybean group, natto made by natto bacillus is a familiar Japanese fermented food although it may not be to everybody's taste. These and other fermentation processes add nutrients and make foods better tasting and easier to digest.

Beyond the use of fermentation to preserve our foods, fermented food is good for our health. To understand this let's go through the process of fermentation. Glucose, protein and carbohydrates in foods are broken down by microorganisms during the fermentation process creating components beneficial for the human body.

The intestines—the part of the body in which I specialize — especially benefit from fermented foods as they help beneficial bacteria to propagate in the intestines. For example, when lactobacillus, which is a typical beneficial bacterium, reaches the intestines, the pH inside the intestines turns acidic thus inhibiting the propagation of bacteria unable to survive in the acidic environment. Many of these bacteria are hazardous; they produce humic substances such as ammonia and hydrogen sulfide, and therefore they are generally referred to as harmful bacteria. By the increased activities of beneficial bacteria, these harmful bacteria lose their power, and the environment in the intestinal tract improves.

The activities of microorganisms are also a vital part of the relationship between the intestines and our immune function. There are various immune cells (such as macrophage, lymphocyte cells, and neutrophils) working in the intestinal tract. They protect the body from pathogens that we may have ingested. Beneficial bacteria, such as lactobacillus, activate these immune cells. This is why our immunity to disease is compromised when the intestines are in poor condition.

Two thirds of the immune cells in our body are concentrated in the intestines, which are the most important part of the digestive tract. When the intestinal environment is disrupted and in a poor condition, the problem goes far beyond the health of the intestines. If nothing is done to improve the intestinal health, the immune power and the life energy of the person will be depleted making them prone to cancers, lifestyle-related diseases, infectious diseases, allergy related disorders and various other problems.

People whose main diet consists of meat, dairy products, and the usual junk foods without any intake of fermented foods require special attention. Over the years in my clinical experience, those people who don't pay attention to the health of the intestinal environment and continue unhealthy diets are the folks most likely to lose energy and stamina and show more and more signs of disease as they age. The merit of daily consumption of fermented foods goes further. Fermented foods are indispensable in replenishing enzymes, which are key to human health. My book *The Enzyme Factor* explains why enzymes are so important and introduces an enzyme-enhancing program I call the Shinya Biozyme, which includes diet, nutrition, and other lifestyle suggestions. I will explain the Shinya Biozyme in more detail in the second part of this book, but it will help you to understand the biology that makes the Biozyme so powerful for your health.

Briefly, enzymes are protein substances, which are involved in all phases of our life activities. It is common knowledge now that they are important in the digestion of foods but they also are involved in breathing, metabolism, elimination and detoxification. Enzymes serve as catalysts for the chemical reactions necessary for living organisms. Their importance may not be fully recognized in modern medicine and nutritional science. It is true, however, that no matter how many nutrients we may get from foods, we would not be able to maintain our energy if we did not have sufficient enzymes in our body. This is why I call enzymes the source of life energy.

We know that there are 3,000–5,000 known varieties of enzymes in the human body. Now, here's the crux of the "microbe factor" for your heath: *The majority of these enzymes are made by intestinal bacteria.* When the intestinal environment is disturbed with the proliferation of so-called harmful bacteria, *the growth of these vital enzymes is impaired.*

Fermented foods contain large quantities of enzymes; therefore you will be supplementing the enzymes in your body by consuming such foods. The enzymes found in fermented foods are digested and absorbed in the body and broken down into peptids and amino acids. It is my theory that these are compounded again as the "miracle" source enzyme, which is the basic substance for other enzymes in our body.

All the work within our intestines by bacteria, enzymes and immune cells to maintain and nourish our health is linked very closely. This is why the key to vitality and head-to-toe health is to improve the intestinal environment. Knowing this, I believe the role of fermented foods is greater than generally recognized. They promote overall health by adding beneficial bacteria to the intestines, boosting the immune system, and making it less likely that we will need to take the extraordinary measure of killing off the "bad" bacteria with antibiotics in order to save the person's life.

In our twenty-first century food production and distribution system, however, much of the traditional benefit of fermentation has been lost. Many of the fermented foods found in supermarkets are fermented for a short time because they are mass-produced, and, in order to make up for this, various additives such as fermentation accelerators, synthetic preservatives, artificial colors, and chemical seasoning agents have been added. Also it is likely pesticides and chemical fertilizers have been used on the food crops. Miso paste or soy sauce mass-produced using soybeans on which large amount of pesticides have been sprayed are fermented foods in name only. You cannot expect health benefits from such foods and consumption of such foods on a daily basis may have an adverse effect on your body.

Actually, "good" and "bad," those value judgments we assign to microscopic organisms, are misleading us. Bacteria are neither good nor bad, they're just part of the natural world. Even those we call "harmful" still have some beneficial roles to play in certain circumstances. In making a space for both good and bad to exist, we will be able to see how the function of our intestines conforms to the way of the natural world.

Unlike bacteria, there is no classification of virus as beneficial or harmful. One may consider that all of them are harmful, in that they threaten the existence of human beings. However, if we simply regard them as "bad," we will see no other solution but to find a way to destroy all viruses, as if nature itself were our enemy. We cannot find our way to health by trying to destroy whole categories of life.

We have developed many medicines such as antibiotics in order to overcome diseases. However we cannot say that this has improved the level of our overall health. Medicines that are chemically synthesized are foreign substances to our body, and therefore they will be in some way toxic. We expect to take medicines when we get sick, and we call ourselves "cured" when the symptoms are suppressed. In approaching our health care in this way we are not considering enough the negative effects that these medicines can exert. Antibiotics, for example, destroy not only the targeted pathogens but also beneficial bacteria. With the activities of beneficial bacteria compromised, the balance of intestinal bacteria is disrupted and the production of enzymes for our immune health is diminished. As a result, the overall level of our health declines.

In order to get out of the vicious circle of a complete dependence on antibiotics to save us from infection, we will have to focus more on strengthening our bodies. One tried-and-true path to physical health is to consume good quality fermented foods that have been known for generations to develop a good intestinal environment, one that elevates immunity.

The link between healthy soil and healthy intestines

We could look at our current agriculture methods in the same way. Our over-reliance on "medication" is found in farming as well. After World War II, farmers in the United States and other developed countries of the world began putting large amounts of chemical fertilizers and pesticides in the soil in an attempt to increase the harvest and improve the efficiency of our agricultural work. Pesticides generally are chemical agents such as insecticides, fungicides and herbicides used to kill insects that eat the leaves and fruits of produce, to kill bacteria that cause plant diseases or to kill weeds.

Today there are about 5,000 registered pesticides. Recently we have prohibited the use of pesticides with high toxicity. Some people believe there is hardly any effect on the human body as long as pesticides are sprayed in moderation. But of course pesticides are chemical drugs that are produced synthetically and they are foreign substances to the human body. Nature is about balance. There is nothing in nature that can be destroyed with upsetting something else. Calling something in nature a "pest" then applying pesticides to kill it will lead to the breakdown of the balance of the ecological system, just as antibiotics break down the balance of our intestinal flora.

Fertilizers are substances necessary for plants and are produced chemically in plants. Nitrogen, which nourishes leaves, phosphate which nourishes fruits and kalium (potassium) which nourishes roots are called the NPK fertilizers (three elements of fertilizers). The components of these chemical fertilizers are absorbed immediately, promising good harvest results in a short time, and thus their use spread rapidly in the U.S. after World War II.

The problem is that a complete dependence on chemical fertilizers will lead to disruption in the mineral balance of soil by the dominance by these three minerals (nitrogen, phosphate and potassium). In nature, there are over 100 minerals. One may argue that deficient minerals could be supplemented, but it would be most difficult to determine the need for each mineral and its proportion to make the soil healthy. Furthermore, there is a problem in that chemical fertilizers are inorganic and therefore they don't nourish microorganisms in soil. As a consequence, dependence on chemical fertilizers leads to the deterioration of the quality of soil, eventually making it difficult to grow produce. It also leads to the deterioration of the quality of the produce grown in this depleted soil. Like the soil it is grown in, the produce will lack the trace minerals found in healthy soil.

We know our daily meals play an important role in improving our intestinal environments. The quality of the produce we eat at those meals is determined by the quality of the soil in which it is grown. There are countless microorganisms coexisting in soil. These soil microorganisms are the key to the life force of the plants.

It is highly likely that heavy use of pesticides and chemical fertilizers is compromising the health of our entire ecosystem, down to and including our own intestines.

Nature, of course, needs no human help to keep the soil fertilized with the right mixture of minerals and microbes to nourish the plants and animals that live off the land.

In autumn, fallen leaves and branches cover the ground. During winter they are decomposed by the work of microorganisms and earthworms in the ground converting the soil into mulch suitable for growing produce. The soil is rich, and loose, with aggregated granules of dirt so that water and air can pass through; it has a soft, fluffy texture. With its abundant trace minerals such as iron, copper, zinc, manganese and so forth, this is an ideal environment for microorganisms to thrive. NPK alone cannot sustain aggregated structures, and food produced from such soil will contain few minerals. According to a report by UN Conference on Environment and Development of 1992 (Earth Summit), the mineral contents of farmlands in various parts of the world have been depleted by 55-85% in the past 100 years.

We can no longer say "Eat your fruits and vegetables to get the vitamins and minerals your body needs." Fruits and vegetables are available in abundance in our country, but they often lack some of the vital nutrients such foods once contained. The organic fertilizers our forefathers used, such as animal dung, fish lees, oil meal, plant ash and so forth, were a rich source of minerals and, when mixed with soil, created a friendly environment for microorganisms. Each of these organic fertilizers is a waste material from the digestion of a living organism, and when returned to the soil, they nourish microorganisms, contributing to the growth of the food we eat. We are part of the cycle of nature, and eating organically fertilized foods puts us in harmony with Mother Nature, rather than at war with her.

The soil in which plants grow functions in the same way as do our intestines. Or, I might say that our intestines are our soil. In both of them, microorganisms called intestinal bacteria or soil bacteria have important roles in maintaining the health of their hosts. The excessive use of chemical fertilizers and pesticides may temporarily increase the harvest contributing to the efficiency of operations, but eventually the soil will become exhausted and turn into an environment not suitable for farming. The same is true with medicines. If you take medicine to cure diseases, you may temporarily eliminate pains and discomfort, but the medicine will also destroy beneficial microorganisms and cause an adverse effect on your "soil" – your intestines.

Due to our limited understanding and pursuit of immediate benefits, we have been destroying our soil and the countless microorganisms which inhabit it. Environmental pollution is nothing but the pollution of microorganisms. All beings in the world are linked together. In so far as we disregard the chain of life, it will be difficult to prevent the deterioration of the soil that sustains our food crops and our own soil, our intestines. The life force of vegetables and fruits and the life force of humans who consume these foods will inevitably deteriorate. As a result, the life force of the ecosystem will deteriorate.

Then, how could we break such a vicious cycle?

I am not an authority on agriculture, but if the environment of the soil has a direct bearing on the environment in our intestines, I would say the key to our health lies in microorganisms. As we have seen, there are countless varieties of microorganisms in the world. The ones we should be focusing on are microorganisms that are capable of improving the health of the soil. For example, there are microorganisms that act upon chemical substances or residual pesticides, helping to break them down and render them harmless. There are microorganisms that prompt the decaying of mulch, and those that curb the work of pathogens. These microorganisms that contribute to the coexistence of human beings and nature are collectively called "effective microorganisms."

Research into ways to combine effective microorganisms for improving soil has been going on for the past century. In an age when modernization has been spreading globally, such a movement has continued to exist although it is quite different from the research that has gone into chemical fertilizers and pesticides with their decisive emphasis on efficiency. Agricultural microbiology studies soil microorganisms and the improvement of soil structure.

It has been proven that microorganisms are effective in purifying water in rivers and deodorizing and composting domestic garbage. They can even be used in the decomposition of dioxin and other toxins as well as in controlling mite and roach populations, which can carry disease and cause allergies. After the Exxon-Valdez oil spill in Alaska in 1989, chemists began to develop bioremedial agents to be used in the second wave of oil spill response. These bioengineered agents enhance the efficiency of naturally occurring bacteria that consume hydrocarbons such as petroleum and spit out carbon dioxide and water.

We still have much to learn about the best ways to work with effective microorganisms. In bringing changes to conventional farming, which since the mid twentieth century has relied heavily on pesticides and chemical fertilizers, we know for sure that effective microorganisms are indispensable in restoring health to our soil.

Farming provides the basis for all human sustenance. We are what we eat, and the nutrients in our "daily bread" are the keys to our health. Farming is the foundation on which the food pyramid rests. If we're going to talk about nutrition, we should begin with a discussion of agriculture.

I have told you that the mineral contents in farmland in various parts of the world have been depleted by 55-85%. The same is true with the mineral contents in vegetables if you compare the vegetables sixty years ago with today's vegetables.

The reason I feel there is a problem with nutritional science in the U.S. is that the quality of vegetables is not addressed and nutritional guidance is based on the premise that all spinach, for example, is equal, nutritionally.

In Japan, however, the Ministry of Education, Culture, Sports, Science and Technology, has kept track of the nutrients in various crops today as compared with crops of years past and published these in the Standard Tables of Food Composition. If we compare the iron content in spinach we will find that it was 13mg per 100g of spinach in 1950 whereas it was only 2mg by 2000. The vitamin C in carrots shows a decline from 10mg to 4mg, and cabbage shows a decline from 80mg to 41mg. Such losses of minerals can be found in many vegetables and fruits.

In the United States, it seems to be assumed that you can get the same nutrients no matter how your food is grown, and it is difficult for farmers to have their produce evaluated for quality. Under such circumstances, it is impossible to provide meaningful nutritional guidance and to restore agriculture in the U.S. As long as we are stuck with the current nutritional science, I am afraid that the nation's food will suffer from a hollowing effect. Personally, I believe the current epidemic of obesity in the U.S. is partially caused by "hollow" food, which leaves the body craving for the health-giving substances that are no longer present in our daily diet.

As a physician I know there is little emphasis or awareness on the part of most doctors as to the effect of diet on their patients' health. Physicians have been trained to prescribe medicines and to rely on expensive tests for diagnosing disease. We can hope that our awareness of the relationship between our bodies, our food chain, and our soil will lead to a change in our approach to modern medicine — away from "warfare" using drugs and chemicals, toward balance and harmony with the world in which we live.

NUTRITIONAL SCIENCE AND ORGANIC FOOD

In the U.S., to be sure, there is an increasing trend toward environmentally friendly farming methods. In organic farming, or natural farming, pesticides and chemical fertilizers are not employed.

In order to call produce "organic," it must be cultivated in soil where pesticides or chemical fertilizers have not been used for three years or more prior to seeding; the farmer must refrain from using prohibited pesticides or chemical fertilizers during the cultivation period; and the farmer cannot use seeds which have been genetically altered. Additionally, foods certified organic have not been processed using synthesized additives or chemicals and the major ingredients of the processed food, excluding water and salt, should contain 95% or more organically grown foods, free from genetic manipulation. With regard to livestock products, the animals must have been fed mainly organic feed, no antibiotics were used and the animals were not subject to genetic manipulation.

It is important, however, not to go for an easy solution and think it is "safe" as long as one is consuming approved organic produce. As I have repeatedly stressed, the issue is how to improve soil, and thus the intestinal environment. I suggest you develop a habit of constantly consulting with your own body. How does your physical condition change by changing your daily intake to environmentally friendly products? Are you feeling lighter than before? Has your health improved? Or, are you experiencing chronic discomfort?

The condition when intestines or soil are energized is a state full of the power of life. It is not easy for us, living in our modern technologically-advanced society, to fully experience the energetic state with which a human being is endowed. Regrettably, the life style of many people continues to lead them further away from their full energetic life force.

We must understand that the food we eat is "life" itself. We take in "life" from fruits and vegetables and transform it into our own life energy. Excessive use of pesticides and chemical fertilizers compromises the life energy available in the vegetables and fruits we eat.

The value of enzymes becomes clear when we start to understand life energy. The reason why nutritional science in the U.S. and Japan fails to sufficiently contribute to our health is because it is missing the concept of "enzyme-replenishing life energy."

Life energy is the spine of our health. In a way, we have exchanged our own life force for a convenient and efficient lifestyle.

The following is a story frequently quoted in Japan. A German physician, Dr. von Bertz, who contributed significantly to establishing modern medicine in Japan, recorded an interesting episode in his diary. When he traveled to Nikko, which is about 65 miles away from Tokyo, he reached the destination by changing horses 6 times and taking 14 hours. His travel companion who used a rickshaw arrived 30 minutes later without switching his rickshaw man. Dr. Bertz was surprised and checked what the rickshaw man had eaten. His meals consisted of balls of brown rice with pickled plumbs, shredded radish pickled in soybean paste, yellow pickled radish and such. He also learned that the rickshaw drivers habitually ate a meager diet consisting of mostly rice, barley, potatoes, millet, and the roots of lilies, with hardly a trace of animal foods.

Dr. Bertz who was studying cutting-edge nutritional science, thought that surely the rickshaw man would have had more strength if he had eaten meat. Thus he hired two rickshaw men in their twenties and provided one with a traditional diet mainly consisting of brown rice and the other with beef. Then he conducted an experiment in which both men were to run rickshaws with a load of 80 kg (176 pounds). The one whose diet was rice balls continued running for three weeks, whereas the one with the diet of meat became too exhausted and had to quit after three days.

If you read history books, you will see countless examples of the power of meager meals among the Japanese. The notion that "meat increases people's stamina" is not based on a proper foundation.

I urge you to be aware of nature's cycles and to learn the link between our intestines and the soil that nourishes our food crops, and between these and the work of microorganisms involved in their growth. Through such efforts, you will be able to see for yourself what the new medical model should be. It should be based on nutritional science, and that nutritional science should be based on a thorough knowledge of enzymes and microbes. Your personal health care model should be based not on a chemical and pharmaceutical war on microbes but on knowledge of an appropriate diet and an appropriate use of supplements. I'll outline my suggestions for how you can improve your health by making peace with nature later in this book, but first it will be helpful for you to know more about how nature works, starting at the cellular level.

Chapter 3

Your Innate Immune System

If human beings as a species are destined to lose the war against microbes, if our path to health and vitality must be by making peace with nature and strengthening our innate immune systems, we will need to know all we can about how these natural systems work.

Happily, medical science has been learning a lot about immunity over the past few years, and one of our discoveries is that we have at least two lines of immune defense — the acquired immunity with which we're most familiar, and a more basic, innate immune system that operates continually to keep us disease-free most of the time, despite the fact that we are exposed to germs every day.

How does this natural defense system work? Let's take an example of a cold. A cold is caused by viruses that are foreign elements to our body. The symptoms we experience, the running nose or sneezing, result from our body's attempt to reject these virus pathogens, but some pathogens will still manage to survive, to threaten the body. At this point white cells kick in. There are varieties of white cells, but the first white cells to react to invading viruses are macrophages or neutrophils. Like Pac-men, these cells literally capture and devour pathogens. Still there are instances when such efforts may fail in getting rid of the cold germs. In such instances, lymph cells come into play to eliminate them. There are two types of lymph cells and they work as a team. First, helper T lymph cells receive information on the structure of the pathogens. This information is then forwarded by macrophages, which issue instructions to B lymph cells to produce antibodies. These antibodies are discharged by B cells like missiles to attach to pathogens to freeze their movements, and, then the "Pac-men" — the macrophages and neutrophils —devour them. In the case of the "common cold" the entire process takes one or two weeks, during which time we suffer the symptoms of depleted energy, sinus and throat inflammation and runny nose. This team effort by lymph cells and others is called the antigen-antibody complex reaction. In this way, we are protected by layers of defense mechanisms.

The functions of antigen-antibody complex reaction are not limited to the removal of invading pathogens, however.

After digesting a pathogen, a macrophage will present the antigen (a molecule, most often a protein found on the surface of the pathogen, used by the immune system for identification) of the pathogen to the corresponding helper T cell.

Once a T cell has recognized its particular antigen on the surface of an aberrant cell, the T cell becomes an activated effector cell, chemical mediators known as lymphokines that stimulate macrophages into a more aggressive form. These activated macrophages can then engulf and digest affected cells much more readily.

Using antibodies, the body stores the information about the structure of the invading pathogen, thus facilitating immune functions if the same pathogen invades the body in the future. The information from the first contraction of the disease is stored for the next generation of antibodies. Each time the same pathogen invades, more antibodies are produced so that the acquired immunity becomes stronger.

This is an excellent system but it is not perfect in that it only responds to the exact same pathogen. Viruses, which mutate very rapidly, can easily adapt to foil it. This is why immunologists have to come up with different flu vaccines every year, and there can never be a vaccine that will prevent the most ubiquitous viral infections we refer to collectively as the "common cold." The system is also slow to go into effect. It takes a few days to a few weeks before antibodies are generated, and thus invading pathogens are not effectively dealt with immediately.

This immune function based on the work of lymphatic cells, called acquired immunity, is definitely a lifesaver, a "high-tech" development of millions of years of vertebrate evolution. In fact, scientists now believe acquired immunity only came into being after the evolution of vertebrate animals with hinged jaws. This does not mean, however, that, during all those millennia prior to the development of vertebrate animals, living organisms did not have immune functions. Living organisms from the earliest stage of evolution must have fought against invaders or have developed ways to coexist with them. The most basic and ancient system is *innate or inherent immunity,* the system that has existed from the earliest stages of evolution, although we are only now discovering how it works. As we have learned more about inherent immunity and how it works, it has become clear that how well this basic immune power is functioning has a great deal to do with the level of one's health.

CELLULAR IMMUNE POWER

We have been focusing on the work of the macrophages and neutrophils. These immune cells, which destroy pathogens by devouring them, may sound primitive when compared to the elegant work of lymph cells, but, in fact, the lymph cells could not do their work without macrophages. In the antigen-antibody complex reaction, unless macrophages present information on pathogens to B cells, antibodies cannot be produced.

At the earliest stages of the evolution of life, however, each single cell would have had to dissolve and dispose of invading foreign elements within that single cell in order to survive. There were no dedicated "Pac-man" immune cells — no macrophages. There would have had to be an immune power even more basic, an immune force inside the cell itself, and it would have had to exist inside every cell from the era when all that existed were single-cell organisms. In fact, it is known that even simple single-cell organisms such as bacteria possess enzyme systems that protect against viral infections. Other basic immune mechanisms evolved in ancient eukaryotes and remain in their modern descendants, such as plants and insects. Since all living organisms today are composed of cells, all human cells must potentially have some innate immunity. Every one of our 60 trillion cells has innate immune power, unless the properties that existed in earlier life forms have been lost somehow. I do not believe this to be the case. I believe that the immune power that existed in primitive cells, or innate immune power, is the real, natural source of our present-day strength, health and life power. This power is what keeps some people from catching colds that sicken others. In short, this earliest immune potential in the basic structure of every living cell is the source of the superior immunity that keeps most of us healthy most of the time, even in the midst of a virtual "sea" of germs.

How do innate immune powers function in each cell? Answers to this question have been emerging from biomedical research only in the past few years. Professor Shizuo Akira and his group at the Immunology Frontier Research Center of Osaka University in Japan have found unique cell sensors called toll-like receptors (TLRs). "Toll" is German for "weird" but also for "fantastic" or "marvelous," and what the TLRs do is marvelous indeed. These receptors catch foreign invaders and secrete antibacterial and antiviral substances. This function is not limited to the cell that has been invaded. By the work of the sensor, other neighboring cells are notified of this danger and all of these cells emit antibacterial and antiviral substances directed at the pathogens. The strong point of their work is the instantaneous response to invading enemies, which allows lymph cells time to efficiently respond to remaining enemies using antibodies. Immune cells such as macrophage and lymph cells commence their operations only after this initial defense mechanism. If the instantaneous defense at the initial stage is efficient, contagious diseases triggered by the invasion of bacteria or viruses are prevented. Furthermore, pathogens that penetrate cells, escaping the attacks of antibacterial and antiviral substances, are faced with the intracellular detoxification. Literally, they are shredded on a molecular level in a process called autophagy. The pathogens are identified inside the cell, bagged and shredded by enzymes.

Reliance on the secondary response with its specialized immune cells becomes necessary only when the innate immune power is not functioning efficiently. As medical science learns more and more about our frontline defense system, we can anticipate we will be able to strengthen it and at last find more completely reliable defenses against flu, the common cold and other viral and bacterial diseases that have long plagued humankind.

The fact that single-cell organisms such as bacteria use enzymes to protect against invading viruses tells us that enzymes are key to our most basic frontline immune response.

Enzymes are catalysts, involved in all the chemical reactions necessary to support life. Even if sufficient nutrients are supplied to your body, these nutrients cannot be digested, absorbed and converted to energy unless enzymes are functioning properly. Enzymes are important for the digestion of the food you eat, but their importance goes far beyond that. They are involved in *all* life activities: breathing, the beating of the heart, the detoxification of the cells, the perception of all external information through the five senses, thinking, responding emotionally and many more.

There are specific enzymes dedicated to each of the life functions. Three thousand to five thousand enzyme types have so far been identified in the human body. The reason for such a huge number is that each one has a particular mission and cannot be replaced by another. Each type of enzyme is unique. For example, in digestion, an enzyme called amylase found in saliva breaks down carbohydrates, pepsin in stomach fluid breaks down protein, and lipase in pancreatic fluid breaks down fat. In the innate immune response, acid hydrolases digest the pathogens inside cells.

Western science has categorized enzymes into two major groups; digestive enzymes and metabolic enzymes, but these limited categories are not necessarily appropriate for today's enzyme research. I would like to depart from such conventional definitions and focus on the work enzymes do inside cells to clean out pathogens and waste materials that would otherwise sap energy from the body.

SANITATION-WORKER ENZYMES

Inside cells, organelles called mitochondria use food nutrients and oxygen to produce ATP (adenosine triphosphate), to provide the energy needed for the various activities of the body. Enzymes inside cells help with this process. Meanwhile, other enzymes inside cells are involved in detoxification. They're like sanitation workers inside the cells where digested nutrients are distributed, working to break down waste and foreign substances. This process is going on all the time in cells all over the body, not just in the digestive tract. These sanitation-worker enzymes clear away the trash so the cells can function normally.

Why is a "sanitation" enzyme so closely linked to human vitality? In order to see clearly the connection, it helps to have a clear understanding of what it means to be fully alive. By understanding this, we begin to more fully appreciate the importance of enzymes, which are at the root of all life activities.

Asian cultures have a name for the life force: The Chinese call it *chi* and the Japanese call it *ki*. Europeans tend to think of the life force as a philosophical concept, but I know it has a scientific basis. A strong life force or *ki* means that the approximately 60 trillion cells in the physical body are actively working. If our cells, which are the basic units of our physical body, are vital then we, who are made of these cells, are also vital. By the same token, if our cells are not functioning well or if something has had an adverse effect on them, we will have a poor physical condition, low energy, and, sooner or later, disease.

Think of it this way: each cell in our bodies is itself a living organism, rather than a "thing." The nutrients from the food we eat and the oxygen from our breath are carried by our blood to all the cells in our body. Each cell has special little organelles called mitochondria containing genetic material and many enzymes important for cell metabolism, including those responsible for the conversion of food to usable energy, in the form of ATP. When ATP is produced smoothly, we are filled with vitality and are able to lead an energetic life.

If a person feels lethargic, lacks motivation or is still tired after a rest, it means that the nutrients taken into the body are not sufficiently transformed into energy in the cells. The person is experiencing ill health or disease. What is the cause for such a poor conversion of food and air to energy? In a word: trash. There is a buildup of waste materials in the cells of the body.

To function well, cells need to be cleaned of the waste materials of energy generation and any foreign elements of pathogens that may have infiltrated. When such processes are operating properly, energy generation will be carried out smoothly and the body will be filled with vitality. However, if detoxification doesn't work smoothly, energy production will be hampered resulting in deterioration of cell activities. Intracellular detoxification, in other words, the clean-up taking place inside each individual cell, plays an important role in invigorating cells for rejuvenation of the body.

Let me explain more about the "sanitation-worker" enzymes involved in intracellular detox.

These enzymes work inside a cell in an organelle called a lysosome. In this organelle, approximately 60 known varieties of enzymes — called lysosome enzymes — are involved in the detoxification process.

The lysosome is actually a microscopic "recycling center" inside each cell. It is surrounded by a membrane, has an acidic interior, and contains hydrolytic enzymes that use water to break down food molecules, especially proteins and other complex molecules. The digested material is then transported across the lysosome's membrane for use in or transport out of the cell. The reason why this recycling is important is because in our cells, the proteins that make up our tissues and organs are constantly being created, and when they are created many defective proteins are also generated. Additional proteins get damaged by radical oxygen, free radicals, or degraded proteins inside the cells. In a process of autophagy, these defective proteins are surrounded by a special saclike film to break them down and dispose of them, while normal proteins are left intact. Lysosome supports such work by creating the enzymes that break down proteins.

Enzymes can decompose defective mitochondria as well as defective proteins. Mitochondria play a central role in generating energy inside cells. There are 500-2,500 mitochondria existing in a cell at any given moment, and they keep dividing. Since such a large number of mitochondria are dividing and increasing, there are naturally numbers of "dropouts" not efficient in their work or whose work is abnormal. When the number of these poor-performing mitochondria increases, the capacity for energy production of cells will deteriorate, and eventually the activities of cells themselves will weaken, or in other words, our vitality will decline. It is the role of the "sanitation" enzymes to surround these poor-performing or aged mitochondria and decompose them. In addition lysosomes generate enzymes to detoxify and break down proteins. There is also a clean up system that is like an "intracellular garbage container" to break down deteriorated enzymes.

Autophagy, the process of digesting nutrients inside the cell, in addition to breaking down defective proteins or misfit mitochondria, supplies energy to the starving cell. In fact, this task of supplying energy is the primary function of autophagy. It functions as a survival strategy when a living being is in a state of starvation because the supply of necessary nutrients is cut off. In such an instance, autophagy is responsible for breaking down nutrients such as protein that are stored within cells and converting them to amino acid, glucose, and fatty acid to supply energy to keep the body functioning until the supplies of nutrients resume.

The reason I call lysosomes the "recycling centers" inside the cells is that in addition to breaking down wastes, lysosomes have the function of recomposing and reutilizing them. And, of course, there are specific enzymes involved. One example is when a baby is born. The newborn is in a sort of starvation state because he or she has moved out of the amniotic fluid and has been cut off from the umbilical chord through which nutrients have been flowing for the past months. As a result, autophagy goes to work to recompose protein and to detoxify cells, keeping the infant alive as he or she makes that stressful transition from the womb into the outside world.

As we saw earlier, autophagy also has the function of surrounding bacteria or viruses, which have penetrated into cells, destroying them and dissolving their remains. In doing so, information is gleaned from the decomposed matter and passed along to be used by the immune functions in the cells, your innate biological defense system.

INTRACELLULAR DETOXIFICATION

There is one huge enzyme that works in a different way, independently of the lysosome and the process of autophagy. This burly sanitation worker enzyme is proteasome and it is the "shredder" within a cell. As the name implies, it marks defective proteins and targets those proteins to break them down, or shred them. This work is referred to as "ubiquitin-proteasome system" and the three scholars who discovered it received the Nobel Prize in Chemistry in 2004. Defective proteins are generated daily inside cells and therefore it is necessary to have a large-scale collective system like the intracellular recycling plant — autophagy — as well as enzymes which are very adaptable in breaking down each defective protein one by one like an intracellular shredder. Simply stated, our cells are using these two functions efficiently so that foreign substances or defective proteins are constantly cleaned out to maintain the health of cells.

Of course, if the intracellular detoxification is not functioning well, the capacity to generate energy by mitochondria gets weaker, causing deterioration of cells leading to the onset of various diseases.

For example, in the midbrain, which handles a part of motor functions within the brain, there is a black spot where a hormone called dopamine is secreted. The reason the area of the midbrain looks black is because mitochondria, which are the energy plants, are concentrated there, and the proteins produced there are known to have high defectivity rates. Unless intracellular shredders are functioning efficiently in this crowded little neighborhood, the mitochondria will become dysfunctional and secretion of dopamine will be impaired, resulting in Parkinson's disease.

Dopamine is known as the hormone in the brain that controls pleasure and motivation, but in this dark spot in the midbrain its main function is to regulate motor functions. The reason why patients with Parkinson's disease have tremors of hands or fingers, muscle rigidity, lack of facial expression, unique disturbance in gait and so forth is the deficiency of the secretion of dopamine there. Also the cause for Alzheimer's dementia is the apoptosis — programmed cell death — of nerve cells from the accumulation of defective protein (amyloid protein). Amyotrophic lateral sclerosis which causes inability of motor nerves to move the muscles of hands, feet, throat, and tongue is the result of defective proteins having accumulated in the brain. The work of the "shredder" enzyme is key to preventing and improving these diseases of brain and nerves in which it becomes difficult to move hands and fingers, to speak freely or chew food. Nor are brain and nerve disorders the only diseases caused by the failure of the functions of intracellular detoxification (autophagy and the "shredders" of the ubiquitin-proteasome system). Evidence is mounting that a problem with intracellular detoxification is involved in immune system diseases, such as cancers and allergies. Focus on intracellular detoxification will be one of the most important developments of medical treatments in the coming years.

While I was researching various functions of intracellular detoxification, I noticed an interesting fact. Similar functions of intracellular detoxification by lysosome are found in plants and microorganisms. The lysosome is an organelle found in the cells of animals including human beings. How does it work in plants? There are organelles in the cells of plants that perform functions similar to the lysosome, and they are the vacuoles.

As the name implies, a vacuole is a sack filled with fluid, and more than 90% of a plant cell is made up of the vacuole with its liquid cell sap. This is why fresh vegetables and fruits are juicy. Many "sanitation worker" enzymes are generated in the vacuole of plant cells, and do their work of intracellular detoxification, decomposing waste matter and hazardous substances.

In recent years, a vacuolar processing enzyme that executes a specific function when infiltrated by a pathogen has been receiving a lot of attention from the medical research community. When pathogens invade a cell, this enzyme is generated in an organelle called a small cystid and goes to work inside the cell's cytoplasm, destroying the membrane of the cytoplasm, thus destroying the infected cell.

This process, called apoptosis, or programmed cell death, sounds threatening, but is actually key to the survival of all living organisms. Insufficient apoptosis results in uncontrolled cell proliferation — cancer. Normally, between 50 billion and 70 billion cells die each day due to apoptosis in the average human adult. This apoptosis process, in which infected cells produce the enzyme that will destroy them, may be considered the ultimate intracellular detoxification.

In a phenomenon unique to plants, numbers of anti-acid components or phytochemicals such as polyphenol eliminate radical oxygen, a free radical, which is generated from waste material or from degenerated proteins. This process of detoxification supports the function of enzymes inside the vacuolar, enabling plants to maintain fresh life power.

There are also toxins in alkaloid categories in the vacuoles of some plants, alkaloids such as cocaine, nicotine, caffeine and so forth. These are created primarily as weapons to fend off enemies from outside, such as pathogens and insects. Plants, being rooted in the ground and unable move around like animals, need a lot of protection. Thus they are packed with "living wisdom" — various strategies to efficiently execute intracellular detoxification.

The life activities of microorganisms are supported by various other sanitation workers, enzymes that assist in the breakdown of toxins. Some types of bacteria, when faced with a danger such as hunger, create copies of themselves (spores), which then digest the original using a secreted enzyme. Thus they choose to live by offering themselves to the spore as nutrients. This may be the original pattern of intracellular detoxification. Fungi, which are eukaryotes and therefore more advanced than bacteria such as yeast or koji bacteria, already have vacuoles inside cells. Of course, similar to plants, intracellular detoxification is performed by the work of enzymes inside these vacuoles.

NEWZYMES

I have a name for all these "sanitation-worker enzymes" which do the work of intracellular detoxification in animals, plants and microorganisms. I like to call them "newzymes" because they are enzymes that help to renew the cells of living organisms. By surveying life activities with the activities of newzymes in mind, you can see the key role enzymes play in the defense of life, health, and rejuvenation.

In order to clarify the functions of newzymes, I will compare them to the digestive enzymes and metabolic enzymes with which people are more familiar. There are differences between them. Remember we said that the digestive enzymes and metabolic enzymes are groups of enzymes which are involved in digesting and absorbing what we eat and converting food to energy in the mitochondria inside cells. Newzymes are a group of enzymes that function when a life is threatened, as opposed to conventional enzymes operating to sustain and support ongoing daily life.

Unless these enzymes are functioning properly inside our cells, our life itself will be threatened. By this way of thinking, you will see that the activity level of newzymes in one's body is literally a barometer to show how high the level of one's life power is. You're only as strong as your newzymes.

Natural immunity is linked to apoptosis wherein those cells that have been infiltrated by viruses or bacteria commit suicide, taking the pathogens with them. When their normal cellular detox fails to defend the cell against invading enemies, the system of self-sacrificing apoptosis is invoked. Broadly speaking, individual cells defend themselves by the complex interactions of three systems; (1) intracellular detoxification, (2) innate immunity, and (3) apoptosis to maintain the energy to keep living. The newzymes, as I call them, are involved in all phases of biological defense and are the "rejuvenating enzymes" encouraging cellular activities.

I want to give more details about the mechanisms of innate immunity and apoptosis where newzymes are involved. I will start with innate immunity. The importance of immune functions is generally recognized, but probably there are still many people who have not heard of "innate immunity." Natural immunity refers to our innate biological defense system. In the past, the focus of medical science has been on the activities of immune cells in blood or lymph fluid. However, this is an acquired immune function created only in the era of vertebrate animals after a long period of progress in evolution and is not universal among all living beings.

The function of these immune cells is referred to as "acquired immunity" in contrast to innate immunity. Acquired immunity recognizes pathogens infiltrating the body as "antigens" and creates "antibodies" thus defending life. It is an immune mechanism *acquired* at the stage when a pathogen infiltrates the body.

Meanwhile, natural or innate immunity has been working in cells all along, since life first developed on earth. Acquired immunity is built upon a foundation of innate immunity. As we learn more about how innate immunity works, the focus of our health care model is beginning to shift. Physicians and others are talking more about the things people can do to boost their innate immunity, with a reliance on vaccinations being secondary and intervention with microbe-killing drugs being our last resort when prevention fails.

Recall the explanation of infectious diseases in chapter 2. We have been troubled with infectious diseases such as influenza, cholera, measles, and the like since the dawn of human history. And yet, needless to say, *not all the people were infected*. Let me put it more accurately. Even when infectious diseases such Spanish flu rampaged all over the world, not all the people were infected and died. While many lives were lost, there were people who were mildly affected or people who were not affected at all. What makes the difference? With acquired immunity, one cannot fight an infectious disease unless antibodies are created by antigen-antibody reaction. It takes a certain period of time to acquire antibodies, and unless one has been infected with the same disease, a new antibody must be created. This is because only one antibody can be effective against one pathogen. In other words, we don't have the ability to take immediate action against an intruding pathogen. What determines life or death with an infectious disease? The answer must lie in innate immunity. Unless the innate immunity, which is innate to all life, is properly functioning, even an acquired immunity cannot be utilized.

In the past, innate immunity often referred to macrophages or neutrophils, which are known for their primitive functions among immune cells. You may not be familiar with macrophages or neutrophils, so I will describe them. These specialized white blood cells are known to devour foreign substances to get rid of them. But they are not primitive cells engaged in devouring only. We know that macrophages have another important function. They act as control centers to issue various instructions to lymphocytes, which destroy pathogens by creating antibodies. Generally, lymphocytes are considered to perform a central role in immune functions, but interestingly they cannot do anything unless they receive instructions from macrophages. Macrophages have a primitive function to devour but at the same time they work to control immune cells.

Macrophages may be compared to a detached force which has taken over the functions of innate immunity working in cells. When single-cell organisms such as bacteria evolved into multicellular organisms and grew in size and complexity, the primary immune function inside cells using intracellular detoxification could no longer defend the body, and thus it is believed macrophage came into being for immune function support.

I want to add a brief comment relating to the evolution of living beings. In the course of evolution to multicellular organisms, the first creature to develop was apparently a digestive tube much like a human intestine. A multicellular organism at an early stage, such as a coral, has only an intestinal tube, and its life is a simple one — to supply nutrients, digest and absorb them in the intestinal tube and excrete.

An intestine is inside a body, but it has regular contact with the outside world through ingestion. Naturally all kinds of pathogens will infiltrate. The reason why ancestors of macrophages (phagocytes) were differentiated from the cells of intestines may have been in order to provide a biological defense against pathogens inside intestines.

Immune cells such as neutrophils and lymphocytes were created by further differentiating from phagocytes, which are the ancestors of macrophages. When we see these developments, the relationship between innate immunity and acquired immunity will become clearer. It may be necessary to temporarily set aside the common knowledge of immunology and to study the innate immune functions of living beings. This is the debate going on at the forefront of immunology.

Apoptosis

Apoptosis is another biological defense system. Apoptosis refers to the breakdown of a cell as the last defense when a cell is filled with an excess amount of foreign substances such as wastes or when a cell is infiltrated by viruses or bacteria too powerful for the cell to defend itself by intracellular detoxification or innate immunity. Apoptosis is referred to as "cell suicide," but it is by no means negative and is a common function among multicellular living things in which it protects other cells from harm. After all, even if it is sacrificed an identical cell will be replacing it. A better way to think of it may be to consider it as a sort of a recycling system.

A good example of apoptosis is when a tadpole becomes a frog; it gets rid of a tail which is no longer useful. Up to a certain stage, the fingers of a human fetus are not differentiated and they look like a web. Cells between fingers gradually go through apoptosis thus forming the fingers of a human hand.

Apoptosis of cancer cells is an important defense strategy. Normally, when cancerous cells are generated in our body, there will be apoptosis of cancer cells to prevent their propagation. However, their activities are inhibited when there are large amounts of radical oxygen and other free radicals which have been generated, turning the body oxidative.

The reason why I recommend that cancer patients follow the Shinya Biozyme in which the intake of animal protein is reduced and the intake of fresh vegetables and fruits is increased is to eliminate free radicals in the body and to induce apoptosis. Of course newzymes are involved in apoptosis. A particularly important enzyme is caspase, which controls the process of apoptosis. These control-type enzymes are kept in a dormant state when they are not required, but upon encountering a situation when apoptosis is needed, another enzyme makes them active. These enzymes are a little different from the enzymes so far discussed but they are similar in that they work when a life is threatened.

THE ADAPTIVE PROPERTIES OF NEWZYMES

Perhaps you are starting to get some idea of the functions of newzymes and how they maintain our lives. The newzymes I envision are groups of enzymes that are involved in cellular detoxification, innate immunity, and apoptosis, the three core lifesaving activities. By activating these enzymes, our cells clean out their own internal waste materials and prevent the infiltration of pathogens. As a result, our life energy flows unimpeded.

The better we understand these newzymes, the more we will know about how to energize them. For instance, newzymes are able to adapt to environments that are different from the environment for digestive enzymes. Newzymes can function well in a mildly acidic environment. When we are healthy, our skin is mildly acidic making it difficult for bacteria to propagate. In an acidic environment, ordinary enzymes cannot fully operate. Therefore such an environment will be the exclusive territory of newzymes, which are able to adjust to mild acidity. Inside the cells, inside the organelles for intracellular detoxification, the lysosomes, the environment is mildly acidic. This acidic environment is a good thing, part of the natural order, because it handicaps bacteria, protecting the individual.

Another characteristic of newzymes is they can function under high temperatures. You may have learned that enzymes are weakened by heat, but that fact applies to ordinary enzymes only. Surprisingly, the properties of newzymes are quite contrary. When you have a high fever from cold, most likely you will lose your appetite. This is because the digestive enzymes are weak under the higher temperature. Digestive enzymes function actively when the body temperature is around 98.6° F, but when the temperature exceeds 100°F or so, the activity level drops drastically. The reason you feel tired or sluggish with a fever may be due to this slacking of activity by metabolic enzymes in the high temperature. Needless to say, activities by viruses and bacteria slow down under high temperatures, and it is the function of newzymes to get rid of them one by one.

Until a few years ago, doctors recommended the fevers be treated with aspirin or other medications to bring the fever down to normal as fast as possible. Now, they're more likely to advise that fevers be allowed to run their course. This is because we're learning that coming down with fever is not abnormal for a body, that it is a normal reaction of the body to get rid of pathogens and to prevent them from spreading. The same is true when tonsils are swollen or when you develop inflammation and fever from an infection of a wound.

Inflammation implies that the area of a wound or infection is mildly acidic. When this happens, newzymes, which can tolerate high temperatures and mild acidity, will be activated to fight against pathogens. It interferes with the functions of newzymes to try to bring down fevers with medications when one has come down with a cold. You could say it is an act against the wisdom of the body's natural order.

SUPPLEMENT NEWZYMES WITH FRUIT

The newzymes are not limited to fighting off infections. They also have the ability to decompose and detoxify every cell in the body. There are 60 varieties of newzymes working in lysosome, which is an organelle inside the cells designed especially for intracellular detoxification. Some of these newzymes are known as competent "decomposers"; they are far superior to ordinary digestive enzymes at decomposing extraneous matter, able to decompose 5,000-10,000 times more. As a group, these newzymes can decompose almost every kind of waste matter, including defective proteins, cell membranes, collagen, fat, polysaccharide and nucleic acid. They are the bulk-decomposing-type enzymes. However, with their superpower decomposing operations, quite a few of them end up destroying themselves. This makes it difficult for us to observe them and we have not found the entire picture as yet. However it is not incorrect to emphasize that newzymes have super powers beyond those of ordinary enzymes because of their ability to decompose waste matter and thus help us maintain health.

Incidentally, it is also the super decomposing operation of newzymes that causes fruits to ripen and increase in sweetness. Fruits have citric acid, which is the source of their sour taste, and they increase in sweetness by a process of fermentation; both the production of citric acid and the fermentation are done by newzymes. They are also involved in the reproduction of fruit. As the fruit ripens, its seeds are likely to fall on the ground. Sometimes seeds or stones are defecated on the ground when animals eat the fruits. From these seeds, new shoots come up and new life begins.

Among these newzymes that are indispensable for fruits to ripen, the enzymes found in pineapples, kiwi fruits, figs, and green papaya are known to be especially superior. In my Biozyme program I recommend eating fruit to supplement newzymes. It is known that these fruit enzymes have a structure that is very close to those of the newzymes working in lysosome. Fruits are a rich source of antioxidant components or phytochemicals to help the function of newzymes. A diet rich in fresh fruit is linked to increasing life power in various ways beyond simply supplementing nutrients. We know that the staple diet of other primates in the wild, like chimpanzees, is built around fruit; it isn't much of stretch to assume there may be a profound relationship between the vitality of all primates – including humans — and raw fruit, rich in newzymes.

WHY IS FASTING LINKED TO LONGEVITY?

One counterintuitive suggestion that has emerged from recent research is that people who eat very, very little may live longer. The studies that suggested this were actually done on other mammals — monkeys, rodents, and dogs — and showed that a diet severely restricted in calories, as long as it still provided adequate nutrition for survival, actually reduced the animals' risk of chronic disease and increased their average life span. It seems to be confirmation of that old saying, "Whatever doesn't kill you makes you stronger."

But does this apply to people? Researchers haven't yet found proof that people who eat very few calories live longer, but they have evidence that calorie restriction in adult men and women causes some of the same metabolic changes that have been observed in the laboratory studies of monkeys and rats. That is, given the proper nutritional balance, calorie restriction in humans decreases metabolic, hormonal, and inflammatory risk factors for diabetes, cardiovascular disease, and possibly cancer. Why is this?

I believe that the class of enzymes I am calling newzymes are the basis for this phenomenon. Because newzymes can adapt to severe environments with mild acidity and high temperature, I have come to regard them as something like special forces, standing by to execute dangerous assignments. These forces are put in motion whenever the organism is faced with a crisis of existence. What are specific cases in our life that pose such a crisis? One would certainly be starvation. Human history has been in large part a fight against starvation. When hunger persists, digestive enzymes or metabolic enzymes that normally work on a daily basis cannot be active. Instead, newzymes in cells go into action.

Even as the organism is under stress and ordinary enzymes in the body are inactive, newzymes are hard at work cleaning up inside the cells of the body. Defective proteins are all decomposed in the process of autophagy and recycled as necessary nutrients for cells. At the same time, wastes and other foreign substances are shredded and cleaned out. With such a process as a daily routine, the cells of the body would stay clean, and, presumably, the vitality of the organism would be stronger than if the newzymes were activated less frequently. We could say that is why people in ancient times who could not get sufficient nutrients like people today were still healthy and able to maintain high life power. They were constantly in a state where newzymes could work actively.

Of course such an environment does not have only positive aspects. When the degree of starvation increases, the stress on body and mind increases and body enzymes are consumed. This, compounded with nutritional deficiency, would have decreased the life span of our ancient ancestors. As a Japanese-American, I am familiar with the history of Japan. Although there were frequent famines in our past, there were many examples of times such as the Edo era in Japan when a peaceful and comfortable way of living lasted for a long time, building a rich culture. And yet, I might say that the Japanese in the past benefited from being unable to eat to their heart's content.

The important thing to learn from this is how active newzymes are. No matter how many years one has added to a lifespan, one cannot live with great vitality unless newzymes are working actively. Is it possible to increase activity level of these vital cell-scrubbers? I believe it is possible. What it will require is a change to a more natural lifestyle, one that involves not always eating to your heart's content.

Perhaps this is not advice anyone wants to hear, but I believe you can increase your vitality by going hungry now and then, so that your newzymes will be activated to clean out and re-energize the cells in your body. Or, simply, eat more moderately, stop eating before you feel full. Or, give up snacking and increase the period of time when you feel hungry within a day. In order to activate newzymes, some moderate fasting will be necessary. I suspect the key to elevating your life power is not in eating, but in *not* eating. Vitality cannot be expressed in numbers such as calories or nutrients, and therefore is very elusive, but it is tied to the work of newzymes inside our cells.

This may be our best anti-aging treatment, a whole new understanding of how to stay vital and youthful. It is time to awaken to the power of newzymes.

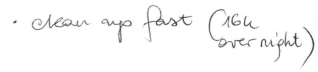

• clean up fast (16h over night)

NEWZYMES ARE ESSENTIAL FOR PREGNANCY AND CHILDBIRTH

We have seen that fasting or eating moderately is linked to the activity of newzymes. There are other crises in our biological life, comparable to starvation. One example is the cycle of fertilization and childbirth. I said earlier that the powerful decomposing activities of newzymes play a part in the process of the ripening of fruit. They are key actors in human reproduction as well. Human reproduction, of course, involves a sperm binding to an egg by penetrating it. This process is facilitated by enzymes. As a sperm comes near an egg, it will eject enzymes from its leading end. Guided by these enzymes, the sperm penetrates and binds to the egg, at which point the enzymes which have led the way to the egg form a film (fertilization membrane) on the surface of the egg cell thus inhibiting the approach to the egg cell by other sperm. There are still unknown areas, but the enzyme that does this penetrating and protecting work may be one of the newzymes.

During the ten months and ten days from conception to delivery, there must be enormous numbers of enzymes involved. Whether all these enzymes should be included in the category of newzymes cannot be determined right away. However, the high amount of consumption of enzymes implies that an enormous amount of life energy is required. Based on what I have stated so far, this stress should stimulate the newzymes to go to work inside the cells, doing their work of intracellular detoxification.

Why do today's women from affluent and technologically advanced societies seem to have more trouble with conception and childbearing than women from poorer backgrounds? Today there seem to be many women who cannot conceive, and miscarriages have increased substantially. Also it has been reported that the sperm count of some men has decreased substantially, and there are increasing numbers of men who have problems with impotence (erectile dysfunction) or infertility (aspermia). As affluence has increased, the birth rate has been declining, and I don't think this is only a matter of changing social values. I strongly suspect that both men and women have lost the vitality necessary for reproduction, and that is where at least part of the problem lies.

Such impaired vitality and fertility, in my opinion, is clearly attributable to the lifestyle of people today who are consuming a diet leading to the deterioration of intestinal features. This diet is based mostly on animal source foods (meat, milk, and milk products), fats, refined grains, white sugar, and junk food. In order to enhance life power and to activate newzymes, which, as we have seen, are involved in the life activities of cells, one must adopt a diet with plant foods and fruits as the base. This is the starting point for everything.

What you eat every day makes your intestinal features better or worse and determines the quality of your blood and cells. I urge pregnant women and the men who are their partners, midwives, obstetricians, and gynecologists to recognize the importance of diet. Nutrition is the base for reproductive health.

THE WAY TO VITALIZE NEWZYMES

The secret to vitalizing newzymes lies in your eating habits; eat less and emphasize fresh vegetables and especially have fresh fruits which are a good source of newzymes. It is important to give yourself an adequate supply of good water.

In addition, it would be good to supplement with the right kinds of nutritional elements in the right amounts to support the work of newzymes. Trace nutrients, vitamins, and minerals are sometimes lacking in our over-processed foods, and you also need antioxidant components such as phytochemicals. The major parts of cells that make up plants are composed of vacuoles containing fluid where newzymes are involved in cellular detoxification. In the fluid, along with the newzymes are supporting antioxidant components or phytochemicals such as polyphenol.

It stands to reason that there are some foods that help induce intracellular detoxification. This, and my half century of seeing the effects of poor nutrition on the human intestines and human health, convince me that a nutritional approach to health care is not only valid, but, in the long run, the only sensible approach.

After all, cells are at the source of all body flows, and newzymes are needed to keep the energy flowing. Going to the source of human health means looking to newzymes for a healthy, youthful, energetic life.

What about enzyme supplements? Most of the enzymes found on the market are ones that support the work of digestive enzymes, and these may be necessary to improve intestinal features and to maintain good physical condition. But medical science is now developing supplements to vitalize newzymes, and supplements of newzymes themselves. Not surprisingly, I am very much interested in this idea, and in the research into various intracellular enzymes. By turning the focus of medical research to cells, which are the basic unit of life, and by focusing on the existence of newzymes working inside cells, we should be able to propose a new way of living that encompasses many human activities — health, longevity, fertility, beauty, our earthly environment and our society. I have great expectations for the developments to come as our understanding approaches the root of life.

Chapter 4

Our Big Experiment in Nutrition and Health

The scientific knowledge about our body's innate immune system that has been emerging over the past few decades has yet to bear fruit in terms of improving the health of people in the twenty-first century. Instead, obesity in the United States has reached dangerous levels, especially among our children, who are coming down with obesity-related diseases not seen in children in the past, such as type 2 diabetes, hypertension, and high cholesterol. Some of this change can be traced to a lack of exercise, especially outdoor exercise, but much of it is related to what and how American families are eating these days. In addition, a growing percentage of American children have allergies. For adults as well as children, auto-immune diseases are on the rise: allergies, asthma, lupus, and rheumatoid arthritis among them.

I see two basic causes for all these food-and-nutrition-related diseases. The first is globalization. Until the past few decades, people mostly stayed in the places where their ancestors lived and ate the things their ancestors grew and ate. Practices of agriculture, fishing, hunting, and food preparation that had been developed over many generations were those that our parents and grandparents relied on still.

Then, during and after World War II, all of that began to change as advances in transportation and communication began to shrink the globe. People traveled more, and so did their food and their technologies for growing, harvesting, and preparing it. This process had been going on in America for two or three hundred years, of course, but even here it has accelerated over the past generation. We've been introducing new varieties of food into our bodies. Almost every local supermarket offers fresh fruits and vegetables from Chili, New Zealand, Mexico and California, even in the middle of winter in the middle of the frozen

Midwestern Great Plains. In any city in the United States you can eat breakfast at a café offering old-fashioned bacon and eggs, lunch at a Japanese sushi place, and dinner at a Mexican taco stand, a fancy French restaurant, or maybe at a Thai or an Ethiopian place.

We love the availability of a variety of foods, but what this means is that our bodies, genetically engineered by nature to eat in a particular way from a particular soil, will inevitably encounter foods our ancestors never ate, foods our bodies aren't equipped to digest easily.

Globalization has also led to another nutritional stressor. Those "fresh" foods from around the globe have been shipped to our local supermarket or favorite restaurant and have arrived looking healthy. In order to pull off this miracle, food growers and processors have developed all sorts of brand-new technologies. They have bred strains of plants that resist bruising and stay fresh-looking as they travel from, say, the orchard in New Zealand to the supermarket in North Dakota. Such plants look great when we buy them, but don't have the taste or the nutritional value of truly fresh fruits and vegetables.

Food growers and processors have made great strides in other ways, too, over the past generation, which leads to the second reason I believe our nutritional health has been compromised by the way we eat today. That reason is that everywhere, from the soil at the farm to the Styrofoam-encased food item we get through the drive-through window, technology has altered the food we eat in ways our bodies often can't handle.

There has been a lot of research into the effects caused by these technologies in recent years. The technologies that have altered our foods include chemical soil fertilizers, soils depleted of micronutrients, genetic seed modification, pesticides, large-scale cage-feeding of livestock, antibiotics fed to and injected into livestock, overuse of animal waste to fertilize soil or to mix with animal feed, and steroids and hormones given to livestock.

Technology has also created a mass-production cuisine all its own, much of it based on corn-based sugars and oils, substances derived from soybeans, processes of sterilization, homogenation, pasteurization, preservatives, artificial fats (such as transfats), artificial sweeteners, and strange new food inventions of every kind. Most of these are at least somewhat digestible for most people, but few are really good for us nutritionally. The result is food that is handy and cheap and sometimes addictively palatable. We have been habituated to eating more and more of these calories that have been emptied of much of their nutrition until we have become a nation of people both overweight and starving for what our bodies really need.

THE JAPANESE EXPERIMENT

Obviously the health of people in the United States has been affected by what and how they're eating, but I can't help thinking of another large-scale nutrition "experiment" that has clearly shown a strong link between nutrition and health. That is the experience of the Japanese people as they began to adopt an Americanized cuisine after World War II.

During the period from 1945 to 1950, a nutritional reform campaign throughout Japan resulted in what has been called the destruction of the traditional Japanese dietary culture.

One of the contributing factors to this destruction may have been the change in the Japanese sense of values triggered by Japan's defeat in the war. It was a psychological shock from which Japanese society emerged with the mentality that their traditional cuisine with its lack of meat had led to their loss in the war. This is the Japan in which I grew up and began my medical studies. Suddenly all things western looked superior to our own traditions. The result was a remarkable change of Japanese diet without parallel in the world, and it wasn't due to this psychological factor alone. There was a deliberate "wheat strategy" by the United States, a winner in the war.

Right after World War II, the disposition of the large amount of surplus agricultural products such as wheat, soybeans, and corn, was an urgent issue on a national level in the United States. The abundant agricultural products, which had been produced to feed soldiers in Europe and Asia during the war, were used in the "Marshall Plan," the postwar European recovery program, and also were consumed in a large volume during the Korean War which broke out in 1950. In the early 1950s, after the completion of the Marshall Plan and the end of the Korean War, the grain surpluses became a problem for the United States. The American farm industry faced plunging prices for their commodities, and a plentiful harvest of wheat throughout the world had a compounding effect on the situation.

To avoid a collapse of American farm prices the government was buying much of this surplus, and the produce that could not be placed in silos and warehouses was piled up on the roads and covered with sheets. Japan, then in the midst of recovery from the war, offered the U.S. a way to unload some of the farm surplus. The U.S. agreed to supply Japan with its surplus agricultural products on good terms: payment would be deferred, and the sales of the surplus to private sectors by Japan could be applied towards Japan's economic rehabilitation.

The agreement included a clause that stipulated that U.S. may use a part of the economic rehabilitation funds to develop markets in Japan for the U.S. agricultural products. The result was the Nutritional Reform Movement which was promoted using kitchen cars throughout the country. Elderly Japanese recall these events. For five years, starting in 1956, kitchen cars, which were large buses that were modified for the purpose, traveled throughout the country to hold outdoor cooking classes. The foods recommended by the Nutritional Reform Movement were the foods of an American-style cuisine — bread made of wheat, meat products, milk, milk products, eggs and fry-cooking using oil or fat. These foods went well with the diet of bread, and encouragement for the consumption of these foods led to the promotion of stock farming, thus opening routes to bring in large amounts of corn and soybeans from the U.S. to feed cattle, and also as the raw material for vegetable oil and corn oil. In fact, Japan is relying on imports from the U.S. for 90% of the cattle feed to date. What the U.S. strategy promoted was a change in the Japanese dietary culture to the type that is convenient for the economic prosperity of U.S.

SCHOOL-PROVIDED LUNCH

This ingenious "wheat strategy" of the United States had another impact on the post-war Japanese dietary culture, and that was because of the free provision of wheat and skim milk powder for school lunches. Nowadays, there are many Japanese schools that serve lunch with rice, but in those days *koppe pan* (bread created in Japan) was the symbol for school-provided lunch. Skim milk powder was initially provided by an American charitable organization as relief supplies, and it should be highly commended because as the result of such aid, some 14 million children throughout the country received the benefits and were spared from malnutrition.

This well-intentioned food relief was to be terminated after Japan's independence in 1951 at the conclusion of a peace treaty signed in San Francisco. However, the United States included a clause in the treaty concerning "provision without charge for school lunch," with an intention to establish a wheat-and-milk dietary lifestyle in Japan. In those days, the school-provided lunch program was facing a crisis, but thanks to this outright gift it was possible to keep it going, and a menu of "bread, milk and a side dish" began to take root in Japan.

Thus, the routine of importing American agricultural products on a permanent basis was established. At the same time, the consumption of rice, which had traditionally been the main ingredient of the Japanese diet, started declining to the extent that a rice acreage reduction policy was enacted. You will see that it is no exaggeration to call this the destruction of Japan's traditional dietary culture.

With this complete change in Japan's dietary culture, the Japanese people became unwitting participants in one of the largest experiments in nutrition and health in the history of humankind. What has been the result of this experiment on the health of the Japanese?

It is true that the Japanese people have grown larger due to the consumption of this diet of milk and milk products that are rich in calcium. When the height of an average Japanese person today is compared to that of the time when I was born (1935), it has increased by almost four inches on average. Young Japanese now have quite different body frames than my generation had. However, to have more height with a better body frame is one thing and to be healthy — free of illness, with physical strength and vitality — is a different matter.

As mentioned in chapter 2, the infant death rate from contagious disease has drastically decreased, and as a result the average life span has reached the rank of first in the world. At the same time, there are 600,000 cancer patients, 16 million people with diabetes including pre-diabetes, 46 million allergy sufferers, and 31 million people with hypertensive diseases, and their population is on the rise. There are increasing numbers of Japanese people suffering from colon cancers, uterine cancer, breast cancer, prostate cancer and so forth, all of which were rare among Japanese before the war.

In Japan where people of my age did not grow up drinking milk, you may think that the number of older Japanese suffering from osteoporosis would be higher when compared to people in the four largest dairy-consuming countries; the United States, Sweden, Denmark and Finland, but that is not the case. Osteoporosis is, as you may know, a disease of fragile bones caused by the deficiency of calcium, and if not treated, will lead to a high risk of bone fracture. Intake of milk is recommended for its prevention

The daily calcium intake by Japanese is said to be about 550mg, twice the amount of intake in 1950. The amount of intake has almost doubled in 60 years, and yet the number of people suffering from osteoporosis is on the rise. People in old days did not drink milk and yet they were sturdier than present day people. They were literally "people with backbones." There are people who say "The average life span was short in those days and that is why there were fewer people who suffered from osteoporosis," and yet, the number of children who break bones from simple falls is increasing as well.

Calcium has more functions than making bones and teeth. A small amount of calcium is found in blood and cells and it contributes to normalizing the functions of a body such as muscles and nerves. Therefore when there is a deficiency of calcium in a body, one tends to become irritable or suffer from mental instability. I will discuss this later on, but this is one of the elements along with excessive intake of refined sugar that is contributing to irritability and lack of emotional control. The problems caused by calcium deficiency are closely tied to the quality of daily diet. In order to make a fundamental change, it is imperative to have a diet which does not depend on animal-source foods and is in line with natural order as advocated in the Shinya Biozyme. One cannot expect any substantial change by simply recommending a balanced diet.

I have written extensively in my Japanese books and in *The Enzyme Factor* about the problems with milk products, especially for the Japanese and other populations not accustomed to consuming dairy. In addition to lactose intolerance, I have observed that there are increasing numbers of patients with intractable colon disorders such as ulcerative colitis or Crohn's disease, and so forth, which were rare 30–40 years ago. It is possible that these incurable diseases may be related to the consumption of animal source foods such as milk, milk products, and meat. The reason for such a speculation is that there have been many cases of symptom improvements after patients changed their diet by refraining from consumption of animal-source food and switching to diets consisting of unrefined grains, vegetables and fruits.

Also there are many cases where those people who had been suffering from allergy diseases such as irritable bowel syndrome, chronic constipation, foul-smelling stool, atopic dermatitis and so forth were given guidance to switch their diet from animal source foods to a diet of mostly plant source and showed gradual improvement in their intestinal features with improvements in their symptoms without resorting to medications.

Cows are herbivores that graze on pasture. But in factory farms they are fed with concentrate feed, including grains and beans which are not their primary diet. In order to induce abundant milk, they are kept in cow pens and are deprived of adequate exercise. In some instances, they are fed with animal-source feed such as fish meal or skim milk powder. In a way, it is same as giving high calorie and high protein food to stay-at-home children. If you put yourself in their position, you would think that you would become sick from such a way of life. In fact, the number of dairy cows that have developed various diseases such as fatty liver, postpartum astasis, mastitis, reproductive disorder, and so forth has been increasing in the past 10–15 years. In particular, displacement of the abomasum, a disease unique to dairy cows, is on the rise.

As many of you may know, cows digest by ruminating and have four stomachs in all. The first three stomachs are supposed to have developed from an esophagus. The first stomach, the largest stomach among them, is known for its function of slowly breaking down grass which is tough to digest, aided by indigenous microorganisms and fermenting. These fermented substances are digested in the fourth stomach, which secretes stomach fluid, and are then carried to intestines. Displacement of the abomasum refers to a symptom of gas buildup in the fourth stomach as the result of indigestion in the first stomach from excessive concentrate feed. Many of these dairy cows lose appetite and refuse to eat. The amount of milk drops and also the animals develop various types of chronic diseases. Often surgery at an early stage is performed to restore the displacement of the fourth stomach to its proper position.

In addition, dairy cows are administered artificial insemination only 60 days after their deliveries, while they are still producing maternal milk.

Presently, with the advancement in the control of livestock, 99% of cows including beef cattle go through the process of artificial insemination, pregnancy and delivery. Artificial insemination is an ordinary process taken for granted by dairy farmers, but I feel we should be questioning whether this is an acceptable practice or not.

The reason for my concern in this issue is that pregnant cows are being milked. We have learned that the milk from pregnant cows (ordinary milk for consumption) contains a large amount of female hormone.

The problem of female hormone of pregnant cows came to light through the research by Mr. Akio Sato, honorary professor of Yamanashi Medical College/University. According to Mr. Sato, when a cow becomes pregnant, the level of the density of female hormone (estrogenic hormone, progestin) in the blood becomes elevated and the hormone migrates to milk. This female hormone is not dissolved during heat sterilization. In other words, a lot of milk on the market contains a considerable amount of female hormone which is far greater than the amount found in milk from non-pregnant cows.

At present, the population which consumes the largest amount of milk is found among children of 7-14 years old, and it is said that each child consumes 320 milliliters of milk including milk products per day. It has been confirmed that milk on the market contains 380 picograms (1 picoram is 1 over 1 trillion grams) of estrone sulfate which is a kind of estrogen. This implies that children before puberty are taking 120 nanograms (120,000 picograms) of estrone sulfate on average. This amount is higher than 40-100 nanograms of the female hormone (estradiol, a kind of estrogen), which is produced by children before puberty. There are some parents who urge their children to consume a quart of milk per day saying "it will make a healthy body." When milk products other than milk, such as cheese, butter, cream, yogurt and so forth are included, the amount of consumption is substantial.

The female hormone contained in milk and milk products is different from the chemical substances that act as hormone, or so-called endocrine disrupters. Because it is a real hormone, its effect on the body is far stronger. In short, by consuming a large amount of milk, which is claimed to be very nutritional and beneficial for the health, children before puberty are given excess amounts of female hormone. Needless to say those children include boys.

What will be the effect of such an excessive female hormone on the minds and bodies of children? Mr. Sato points out that these children of the baby boomers are the first generation in Japan who have been fed with milk even before their birth (through their mothers) and that they have much lower capacity for reproduction. For example, the pregnancy rate of childbearing age (15–45) in 2004, when the second-generation baby boomers were in their twenties, shows 50% decline when compared to the rate in 1973, some 30 years earlier. We cannot account for such a change by simply attributing to changes in concept of values or to late marriages. In fact, there is an unusual problem of infertility or oligospermia. Milk may not be the only cause for all these problems, but we cannot deny that the western style diet including milk has had an impact on the decline in fertility.

Furthermore, breast cancers, prostate cancers, ovarian cancers, uterine cancers and so forth in advanced countries have been increasing after 1940-50 when large consumption of milk and milk products started. Through counseling patients battling breast cancer or prostate cancer, I have confirmed that those patients had consumed milk, cheese, yogurt, and so forth on a daily basis.

I think that present day nutritional science, which was conceived within the constraints of the post-war world, is due for an overhaul. On my part, I have devised Shinya Biozyme, which is based on up-to-date enzyme nutriology. I am recommending this method to many people, including patients who visit my clinic. I believe that it is time to establish a new nutritional science from a viewpoint of the health for each person, completely free from the economic interests of food manufacturers.

Your body is designed to stay healthy and vital by cleaning its cells naturally, using your rejuvenating enzymes, your newzymes. The Biozyme method works with these newzymes, of which there are as many as 60 trillion inside your cells. Once you understand how to awaken these enzymes, you can enjoy increased vitality and ageless years.

Part Two

THE SHINYA BIOZYME

Chapter 5

Rejuvenate on the Cellular Level

You can maximize your *ki,* your energy for life, and you can do this by helping your body function in the way nature intended it to.

Having increased vigor does not involve using vitamin pills or energy drinks. It does not involve artificial stimulants to give a quick boost to a tired body. Rather, you can release your body's natural vitality internally, at the very level of your cells.

Vitality is the key to health and beauty, as well as energy, and, in the long term, you cannot have vitality while eating poorly, no matter how many stimulants and supplements you take. To elevate your life power, you will need to improve your body's natural intracellular detoxification. The Shinya Biozyme will show you how to make this an easy practice in your daily life.

Our body consists of 40–60 trillion cells. When each of these cells is actively working, we have youthful vitality and health. If something is interfering with the functioning inside the cells, we lose energy and become more vulnerable to disease. Inside cells, there are organelles called mitochondria which produce energy for our activities. The oxygen we absorb from the food nutrients we eat and the oxygen we breathe are carried to these mitochondria and are converted to energy. In active, healthy cells, the energy conversion by mitochondria is functioning well. As long as these good conditions continue, we can stay active and motivated, regardless of age. Declining vitality implies that something is hindering the activities of mitochondria in our cells. I call this something cell garbage. In order to restore the health of our cells, it is necessary to clean out the garbage through the body's natural process of intracellular detoxification.

CLEAN OUT THE GARBAGE IN YOUR CELLS

If you feel tired when you get up in the morning it may mean you have a large amount of garbage in your cells. Unless such garbage is removed, cells will not function well. You may try to be active but will find it difficult. If our brain cells contain a large amount of garbage it could lead to the onset of dementia and Alzheimers disease, or trigger a stroke.

Garbage in the cells will lead to the aging of cells, cells that are not repaired, and an immune system that can not function well. We may become prone to infectious diseases or to an onset of cancer. Since the body is made of cells, the inferior activities of cells will impact the health of the whole body.

DEFECTIVE PROTEIN IN CELLS

The majority of the garbage in our cells is nothing but useless defective protein. The nutrients we get from food are digested and absorbed in our intestines and are carried to all the cells through the blood. Protein is one of these nutrients and is dissolved into amino acid in the small intestine and then is converted to new protein in our cells. The process of synthesizing this new protein can produce a large amount of garbage as defective protein. A diet composed of mostly animal-based foods (meat, cow milk and milk products) is the major cause for this production of garbage protein. Many people carry large amounts of this trash material, which has not been decomposed sufficiently in the cells.

Unless it is removed properly, the intracellular constipation will remain. The deterioration of metabolism as one gets older is due to intracellular garbage, but it is wrong to attribute this simply to aging. If proper care is taken with diet and other lifestyle factors, you can remain energetic despite advancing age.

So what should we do to clean up the garbage inside our cells?

There is a dedicated detoxification system inside our cells. The newzymes, those rejuvenating enzymes discussed earlier, are involved in this detoxification system. Depending on the level of activities of these enzymes, the intracellular garbage is removed and is even recycled.

Recall the discussion in chapter 3 about how autophagy operates inside the cells with:

1. intracellular shredders
2. recycling plants
3. intracellular waste bins.

1 AUTOPHAGY   FASTING

Not eating is the key to turning on autophagy, which is the body's intracellular recycling plant. Recent research has suggested that there is a simple mechanism to activate this recycling plant in your system.

When your body is faced with the possibility of starvation it activates autophagy. As discussed in chapter 3, Prof. Noboru Mizushima of the Tokyo Medical School has presented research on exactly how and why this works. By simulating a short state of starvation you switch on autophagy, your body's garbage recycling plant. Nutrients from foods we eat are absorbed from our intestines and carried by our red blood cells to cells throughout the body. A state of starvation implies that the flow of nutrients from intestines through the blood to 60 trillion cells stops. In traditional nutritional science, it was considered important to get necessary nutrients in good balance so that one would not face a state of starvation. With this premise, one is expected to take three meals punctually to supply a minimum amount of calories for daily activities. However, with such a dietary practice autophagy, the process of detoxifying inside our cells, probably cannot function adequately and, if so, an increasing amount of garbage would build up inside our cells.

NEW PROTEINS ARE SYNTHESIZED
FROM GARBAGE PROTEINS

Science is just beginning to become aware of and to try to understand protien recycling. When we think about it, we know that one can survive for a very long time without food if one has water. The reason for this is that the recycling plants within our cells are activated and new proteins are synthesized from defective or "garbage" proteins. In other words, when one is not eating, regeneration of tissues can still go on. Furthermore, the inventory of defective proteins is used up, wiped out during this process of synthesis, thus promoting detoxification inside cells and making cells more active.

MIRACLE OF AUTOPHAGY

Of course if the state of starvation continues there will eventually be no more material for recycling and the body will devour its healthy cells leading ultimately to death. What then is the definition of a "reasonable" state of starvation? We evolved as humans through a history of struggle against starvation. Even under stressful circumstances we have been able to survive and to prosper. The recent findings of biological science help us understand why this struggle for survival was successful. Our own body's ability, in the face of starvation, to recycle protein through the process of autophagy is the miracle that turned the tide in our favor. When our body is in a state of starvation, excess garbage in our cells is cleaned out and recycled into new protein that is turned by the mitochondria into energy. Through the experience of starvation, a kind of power from necessity was unleashed.

By glutting ourselves with foods, we have deprived ourselves of the activities of our rejuvenating enzymes, keeping our body's recycling plant from operating.

What the Shinya Biozyme teaches is that cellular detoxification is as much about when *not* to eat as it is about how to eat. Autophagy is activated when the body thinks it is in a state of starvation. It is within our means to safely and easily mimic such a state by employing a technique I call the "Little Fast." The purpose of this kind of fasting is not to suppress the calorie intake or to reduce excess body fat. Our purpose is to activate rejuvenating enzymes by temporarily inducing a simulated state of starvation as a means for intracellular detoxification.

Chapter 6

The Shinya Little Fast

1. The Shinya Little Fast is a breakfast fast, but the starting point of the fast is not the morning of the fast; it starts the night before. In order to reduce the burden on the stomach and the intestines and to conserve your body's enzymes, have dinner no later than 6 or 7 P.M. the night before your breakfast fast. After dinner and prior to going to bed, nothing should be consumed except for good water. I define good water as water that has been purified of chemicals like chlorine and other toxins and that has a pH around 8.5. I myself drink Kangen water, but you may choose your own filtered water or mineral water. Drink the water at room temperature because cold water will lower your body temperature and your immune strength.

2. Upon rising the next morning drink two to four cups of room-temperature water. Twenty minutes or so later, eat a little bit of fresh organic fruit. You can substitute fresh enzyme juice for the fruit if you like, but do not eat any other food until lunchtime.

   Fresh enzyme juice : *Spinach or arugula mixed in a blender with a bit of apple and a squeeze of lemon juice makes a very satisfying fresh enzyme juice.*

3. Drink two to four cups of water before noon. You may sip from a bottle several times or you may drink it all 30 minutes before lunch.

If you had dinner the previous night at 7 P.M. and you don't eat anything but a little fruit until lunch at noon the next day you will have fasted for about 17 hours. You have fasted more than half a day by simply adjusting your breakfast. In other words, half a day is spent fasting to activate intracellular detoxification. Necessary nutrients will be consumed during the rest of the day.

The Shinya Little Fast lessens the burden on the stomach and intestines while maximizing their activities. I would not suggest making the Little Fast a daily practice, but by repeating this method periodically, your cells will recover in a short period of time and you will be freed from fatigue of body and mind and will have new zest in your life and work. You will notice that this is not a difficult method at all.

FRUIT AS PART OF THE FAST

You may have a concern about consuming fruits, which can contain high amounts of sugar. We are suggesting only fresh fruits, eaten raw, without any heat applied. The reason fresh fruits are recommended during fasting is that they can be absorbed without the help of digestive enzymes and so impose no burden on the stomach and intestines. Furthermore, fresh fruits contain enzymes that are the source of life energy as well as minerals and vitamins to help those enzymes. Excessive consumption should be avoided, but a reasonable amount of fruit assists the effect of the Shinya Little Fast.

AN AGREEABLE SENSE OF HUNGER

If you feel hungry, it is an indication that the autophagy, or intracellular recycling plant is operating and detoxification is in progress. The primary objective of fasting is to intentionally create such a state of hunger. Some people are constantly chewing gum or eating candies, chocolate, etc. You should refrain from such a habit during the 15-17 hours of the Little Fast so that you experience the sense of an empty stomach.

The important point of the Little Fast is not necessarily to fast at breakfast. The point is to simulate a state of starvation so that autophagy (cellular detoxification) can kick in. If you fully understand this, you may change the time of day to suit your own convenience. I am suggesting the Little Fast at breakfast, but if you can be satisfied at dinner with a little fruit or an enzyme drink, it is quite all right to fast at dinner and then to have a hearty breakfast. The whole idea is to provide a time to feel hungry. When you feel hungry, you may have the impulse to satisfy the hunger immediately by eating. Instead, cultivate the idea that a little hunger is a good thing and be willing to just experience it for a little bit. Hunger means that intracellular detoxification has kicked in and your rejuvenating enzymes have started working. The important point in the Shinya Little Fast is to accept hunger with a positive attitude. Through an agreeable sense of hunger, your body will experience cellular rejuvenation. *Remember, we are not refraining from eating to reduce calorie intake but rather to understand and practice the rejuvenating benefits of rational fasting.*

THREE GROUPS OF NUTRIENTS FOR FASTING

Shinya fasting is not food deprivation. There are nutrients you must get during the fasting period. In proper fasting, it is very important to eat better rather than reduce the amount of intake. It may be necessary to put aside the traditional nutritional knowledge you have learned and to consider the new nutriology I have explained. This is the base for the Shinya Biozyme and is aimed at elevating the health of your intestines and cells. The Shinya Biozyme classifies nutrients into the following 4 groups: A – water and enzymes, B – minerals and vitamins, C – phytochemicals and dietary fibers, and D – carbohydrates, proteins and fats.

The nutrients that should be aggressively supplemented during fasting are those in groups A through C. To put it in another way, fasting implies refraining from nutrients in the D group (carbohydrates, proteins, fats), which would be converted to energy, and taking in nutrients of groups A through C, which contribute to the work of respective organs and promote intracellular detoxification. The reason why I recommend dinking water and eating fresh fruits or enzyme juice in the morning is that they supply nutrients A through C efficiently.

FAST – ABC water
minerals
phytochemicals

CHEW YOUR FOOD

At lunch and dinner try to increase the number of times you chew your food, because this will help digestion and absorption by the intestines and you will not feel as hungry. Some say they feel weak unless they eat breakfast, but if you stick to the above, your body will gradually adjust. When you feel comfortable with a sense of hunger, it is proof that your recycling plant is functioning. Sensitive people may actually feel their body conditions improving. Some find that the puffiness of their faces or limbs disappears as their cellular function improves. Some may pass hard stools or a large amount of stool despite a small intake of food as the intestines become more active and get rid of impaction. Body weight and body fat may come down, bringing cholesterol, uric acid and blood glucose levels to normal values. By rejuvenating cells, your body condition improves naturally, restoring vitality.

SHINYA LITTLE FAST IS NOT A WEIGHT-LOSS DIET

Remember, the Shinya Little Fast is not a weight-loss diet. This style of fasting cleans garbage inside cells to restore their most energetic function and to activate the movement of the intestines for smooth evacuation. Weight loss is merely one of the possible results of such an internal reform. When people with metabolic syndrome or insulin resistance go on a diet restricting calorie intake or increase their exercise, they may lose weight and body fat for a while, but they end up regaining the weight because they are not detoxifying at the cellular level.

Chapter 7

The Four Groups of Nutrients in the Shinya Biozyme

THE SHINYA BIOZYME CLASSIFIES NUTRIENTS INTO THE FOLLOWING 4 GROUPS:

GROUP A   Water and enzymes
GROUP B   Minerals and vitamins
GROUP C   Phytochemicals and dietary fibers
GROUP D   Carbohydrates, proteins and fats

WHY CAN ONE SUFFER FROM MALNUTRITION DESPITE SATIATION?

Take a look at the nutrients in A through D again. Many people who have opulent meals are still deficient in nutrition. A diet of animal-based food (meat, cow milk and dairy products) and refined grains (white rice, bread, pasta) may be severely deficient in nutrients in groups A through C. Many of those who think they are eating enough vegetables may still be deficient in enzymes because they are not consuming raw vegetables. Enzymes in vegetables can be compromised or destroyed by cooking.

CHOOSE FOOD WITH LIFE POWER

Many of the foods we eat are deficient in nutrients and have little life power. It is the life energy in the food that counts. Many of the current methods for cultivating crops and processing our foods today have combined to strip them of their life power. What soil was the food grown in? Was it sprayed with pesticides? Was it transported a long distance?

Was it genetically modified not for its nutritional value but for its ability to survive shipment and storage?

CHOOSE WHOLE GRAINS

Eat brown rice and whole grains. Refined flour and white rice are missing the germ and the bran, and you cannot get enough Group B minerals and vitamins from such rice and flour. After a meal of white rice or bread or pasta made from refined grains, the body's glucose level elevates, upsetting one's metabolic balance and stressing the system. Reducing calorie intake is meaningless when the quality of food you *do* eat is ignored.

MINIMIZE THE CONSUMPTION OF FOODS THAT GENERATE GARBAGE IN YOUR CELLS

Physical disorders such as headaches, stiff shoulder, constipation, diarrhea, edema, chills, menstrual disorders, and allergies can be the result of cellular garbage accumulated over a long time. To change this negative cycle, gradually change your diet to reduce the consumption of animal-based foods and refined grains, which generate garbage in the cells. I suggest you begin such a change with a small step that is relatively easy for you to take without stressing yourself. Health is not about denying the pleasure of your meals but rather about forming a new practice for a more energetic life. I hope you will digest the nutritional principles I explain and accept at least some of my suggestions enthusiastically. Then you will be able to feel the positive changes. Start with what is possible for you, and this success will build upon itself to restore healthy function to your cells and vitality to your spirit.

Many think that meat and dairy products are more nutritious than plant foods such as vegetables and fruits, but I disagree. Animal-based foods contain animal fat and cholesterol that are hazardous to our bodies if taken in excess. Also they lack dietary fiber and thus their consumption may lead to deterioration of intestinal features by generating toxic substances and propagating vast amounts of bad bacteria.

- Make friends with a temporary sense of hunger
- Consume plentiful trace minerals and vitamins *whole grains*
- Cut back on eating meat products, cow milk, and dairy products, which are burdensome to your intestines.

The nutritional science of today does not understand what their so-called balanced diet, which includes meat and dairy, does to the walls of the intestines and ultimately to the health. I find it difficult to understand what is meant by "balanced" in such an approach to nutrition. What kind of diet should we follow for true balance? What diet would lead to an improvement of intestinal features?

THE RATIO OF PLANT-BASED FOOD AND ANIMAL-BASED FOOD SHOULD BE 7 TO 1

To start with, I would like everyone to become aware of the problems posed by our belief in the benefits of eating meat. Eating meat does induce growth, but this does not mean that one will not grow unless he eats meat. Take a look at wild animals for example. Herbivorous elephants, bulls, horses and so forth are well built and have more developed muscles than carnivorous animals.

Carnivorous animals, such as lions or cheetahs, are known for their instantaneous power to capture prey, but they don't have sustained power. Herbivorous animals are by far superior to lions and cheetahs in stamina. We cannot come to a categorical conclusion that meat-eaters are naturally stronger or have better body constitution.

As humans are we carnivorous or herbivorous? Generally we are categorized as omnivorous, but this is not necessarily correct. The diet of chimpanzees in the wild consists of about 50% fruits, about 45% other plants (roots, leaves, root vegetables) and about 5% insects (ants, etc.). They maintain their health with an almost totally vegetarian diet. In view of the natural order, the diet of our closest relative, the chimpanzee, may serve as an idea of what the human diet should be.

The examination of the teeth of various animals reveals interesting results. The teeth of carnivorous animals are mostly canine teeth and herbivorous animals have mostly molar teeth and incisors. Human teeth have the ratio of five molar teeth to every two incisors and one canine tooth. Generally, molar teeth (back teeth) are for grinding up grains and beans, and incisors are for biting into vegetables and fruits, while canines are for tearing meat. If we take this into consideration, a balanced meal would be five parts grains and beans, two parts of vegetables and fruits, and one part of meat and fish and/or shellfish.

Based on the above information and my own years of clinical experience, I have come to the conclusion that a diet of 7 to 1 ratio of plant-based food and animal-based food (about 85% and 15% respectively) is the ideal balance to conform to the natural order. Of course we know that meats have adverse effects on intestinal features and therefore it will be advisable to eat fish as animal-source food. At any rate, you will agree that, based on this idea of balance, most people today are consuming too much animal-source food. This is against the natural order and that is why we have come to suffer from various diseases. This is the fundamental problem with the typical American meal.

My experience in both the U.S. and Japan has led me to develop the Shinya Biozyme. I call it Biozyme, combining bio- and enzyme, because the diet elevates vitality by prompting the activities of enzymes in the body. The key to the diet is 85% plant-based foods plus 15% animal-based foods.

Fifty percent of the 85% plant-source foods should be unrefined grains and cereals. Refined (white) wheat and white rice start out as whole grains and brown rice, and then the germ and bran are removed by milling machines. The unrefined grain in the Biozyme diet is unrefined

brown rice /pasta /bread

whole wheat and brown rice. Simply switch the white breads, pasta and white rice already in your diet to organic whole grains and brown rice and you have taken the first step in improving your intestinal features.

How does brown rice lead to better health? First of all rice is the seed of the rice plant. Brown rice is actually the seed after its outer chaff is removed. Brown rice is composed of the germ which is the plant embryo from which a new plant would emerge, the bran which includes layers of fibrous tissue with protein, vitamins, minerals and oil, and the white endosperm which is an energy source used by the germinating rice plant. In other words, to consume brown rice is to receive the life power of the rice plant. White rice, on the other hand, is rice after both bran and germ or, if we think about it, the life force, has been removed. In other words, it is a dead food. Eighty percent of the nutrients of rice, such as vitamin B_1, vitamin E, iron, phosphorus, calcium, magnesium, and dietary fiber, are concentrated in the germ and the bran. The only nutrients remaining in white rice after the milling process has removed the germ and the bran are from the endosperm. The endosperm is primarily carbohydrate, because it is an energy source in the plant for the germ and the bran. You may feel full from eating white rice, but you will not be promoting your life power.

PROBLEMS STEMMING FROM REFINING GRAIN

Clearly, the white rice we are eating is dead food that has lost most of its major nutrients in the milling process. Japan designated white rice as the official rice after World War II and at the same time accepted the American wheat strategy and aggressively promoted bread made from white flour for school lunch programs. The rice that people ate in a traditional Japanese diet was partially refined by removing a portion of bran or was sprouted rice, which had the germ but not the bran. By switching to white rice, the drop in the power of rice as a staple food was inevitable. During this time, even white rice was becoming unpopular in Japan. At one point a famous Japanese university professor published a best-selling book, the title of which would translate into English as *Eat Rice and You Will Turn Into an Idiot.* The consumption of rice gradually declined to the point where a rice acreage reduction policy was enacted in the 1970s.

As for the bread, which was replacing rice in Japan during this time, major nutrients were missing because it was made from flour produced by refining wheat, thereby removing the germ and the bran, which, as in rice, contain the majority of the nutrients. Furthermore, numbers of additives were employed during the process of kneading and baking in order to stabilize fermentation and promote longer shelf life. It is not difficult to conclude that the prevalence of bread, which has overtaken even white rice as a staple in Japan, has contributed to the decline of the vitality of the Japanese. For Americans, who for years embraced refined flours and grains, an epidemic of obesity has awakened awareness of the damage done to health by the unsatisfying calories in refined carbohydrates.

In addition to destroying the nutrient value by refining grain there is also the problem of oxidation. With regard to white rice, the process of oxidation takes place rapidly, since its skin or bran has been removed. White rice is prone to damage when compared to brown rice, and it loses its robust taste. Japanese people prefer new crops of rice, because oxidation destroys the taste when rice is stored in a warehouse for a long time. To put it another way, we are refining rice to lower its taste as well as its quality.

Even when we try to replace the nutrients destroyed in milling, it is difficult to replenish trace nutrients such as vitamins and minerals. vitamin B_1, for example, is indispensable for converting carbohydrates to energy. When we cannot get enough B_1 from our daily diet our energy metabolism is compromised and we will be prone to symptoms of deficiency such as tiring easily or a swollen body. Carbohydrates are the source of energy for our brains and nerves, and therefore a vitamin B_1 deficiency will result in an attention deficit and irritability.

We know now that this deficiency is cured relatively easily by supplementing foods containing vitamin B_1 such as brown rice. Of course if nothing is done, our neuronal system will be impaired, causing numbness of hands and feet and functional deterioration of the heart. It has been pointed out that such symptoms are identical to the symptoms of beriberi, which used to be Japan's national affliction along with tuberculosis before the war. Beriberi is caused by vitamin B_1 deficiency. During the prewar era, Japan was becoming affluent and rich people in cities were switching their main diet to white rice. It is said that this accounted for the increasing number of people suffering from beriberi among the affluent in cities in those days. There was hardly anyone suffering from it in farming villages and thus beriberi was called the sickness of Edo, named for that affluent pre-modern period in Japanese history.

Also in the Meiji era in Japan, there was a problem of beriberi spreading among soldiers and sailors. The Japanese navy took measures by switching the diet from rice to rice mixed with barley containing vitamin B_1 and succeeded in eliminating the disease completely. On the other hand, the Japanese army believed that the disease was brought on by bacteria. Rintaro Mori (known for his pen name of Ogai Mori) was the Surgeon General and he refused the introduction of rice mixed with barley. The result was that there were 250,000 beriberi patients during the Russo-Japanese War of whom 28,000 soldiers died. The total death toll of the Russo-Japanese War was 47,000.

THE MEANING OF EATING WHOLE FOODS

Beriberi was again prevalent in Japan a decade ago, and people today, whose diet includes white rice, white bread and pastries may be affected by vitamin B_1 deficiency. When you see youngsters who are restless and are quick to lose control one might imagine that this so-called Attention Deficit Disorder might be caused by a chronic vitamin B_1 deficiency. Problems are also caused by excess intake of refined sugar and caffeine which I will cover shortly, meat, milk and milk products, bad quality plant fat such as trans-fatty acid, and chronic vitamin B_1 deficiency caused by the over-processing of grains.

Vitamin B_1 is found in pork, liver, beans and so forth, but, as mentioned earlier, the benefits of getting vitamin B_1 from meat are more than offset by the problems. The rice with barley mentioned earlier has been known as health food from the old days because the deficiency of vitamin B_1 in white rice is supplied by barley. If one eats brown rice, the nutrient is already there, right in the rice. Isn't it a weird idea to remove the nutrient and then to supplement it with other food? If you mix barley with *brown* rice, the values of the nutrients as well as the life power will be much higher. Barley is hard and difficult to cook, and therefore it is common to remove the outer skin and steam heat and flatten it with a roller for cooking purposes. Barley contains more calcium and dietary fibers than brown rice and therefore the combination of brown rice and barley is very effective for nutritional support.

There are other grains such as amaranth, red rice, which is also called ancient rice, and black rice, and these contain abundant nutrients — vitamins, minerals, essential amino acid and so forth. Beans such as soybeans, red beans, kidney beans, and black beans are also a rich source of plant protein, calcium, vitamin B_1, and dietary fibers. These grains and beans are getting attention as health foods because they are whole foods, which we consume as a whole, including their seeds, which are the source for life power.

When we are busy with our modern convenient lifestyle it is easy to forget we are receiving energy from food to nourish our life. The concept of analyzing all foods by breaking down respective nutrients and calories may sound rational, but such an attitude can lead to a misunderstanding of life power. Some people believe that the important point is how many nutrients one can absorb from a food whether it is a whole food or not, but I must say that patching parts together will not create a whole. In this respect, a whole food seems to work much better than just supplementing dead foods with vitamin and mineral nutrients.

Our ancestors adopted whole foods in the form of grains. Convenience for their storage may account for the selection but I believe there was another purpose, which was to receive life condensed in grains. As for myself, I eat brown rice mixed with multiple numbers of other grains such as flattened barley and amaranth. Needless to say, this is a source of health and wellbeing.

NUTRITIONAL SCIENCE PRODUCES PEOPLE WITH DIABETES

As people in the United States seek to eat a healthier diet, many will favor rice over bread and potatoes, but, actually, white rice is no better for you than white bread. Again, Japan, where many people eat white rice as a staple food, provides an example of what NOT to eat. White rice is easier to eat because it is refined, so it can be digested and absorbed by the body immediately, but this poses a problem of elevated glucose level after a meal. Carbohydrate, which is the main component of white rice, is converted to glucose during a digestive and absorptive process and becomes the source of energy for daily activities. The excess glucose is sent to the liver through the blood and stored as glycogen. When energy is required, the glycogen is converted back to glucose and sent to cells of the entire body through blood and converted to energy by mitochondria in cells.

The so-called glucose level refers to the density of glucose in blood, and when such a level exceeds the normal range, one will be diagnosed as diabetic. The glucose level is regulated by a hormone called insulin, which is excreted by the pancreas. When one consumes too much food loaded with carbohydrates, whether white rice, bread or pasta made from refined wheat flour, corn, potatoes, fruits, or white sugar, insulin will not work adequately and carbohydrate energy will not be distributed throughout the body. Consequently the person usually feels tired, and *is* tired, all the way down to the cellular level. Symptoms, beyond the tired feeling are sluggishness, excessive thirst, and an inability to concentrate. There are two types of causes for poor insulin function (1) impaired insulin secretion from the pancreas and (2) insulin resistance. In both cases, problems of energy metabolism are greatly influenced by overeating and/or the lack of exercise.

There are many diets prescribed for the prevention and control of diabetes that are not producing results. Often, a diet with balanced nutrition consisting of grains, vegetables and meat is recommended. As I mentioned, refined grains are not "balanced" nutritionally. White rice might be less hazardous to the blood sugar levels than bread or pasta made of refined wheat flour, but still it tends to cause excess secretion of insulin. Also its nutrients have been removed from refining and therefore it is necessary to include various types of foods to prepare a meal that is nutritionally well-balanced. Sometime ago, the Japanese Ministry of Health, Labor and Welfare advocated 30 different foods per day, but I wonder how many people really followed such a practice. Adherence to white rice is nothing but the bad tradition promoted by the nutritional science in post-war Japan, just like the promotion of "enriched" white bread in the post-war United States.

If you are concerned over elevated blood glucose, I suggest you switch to whole grains or mixed multiple grains which are a rich source of dietary fibers and are digested slowly. Such a diet prevents a rapid elevation of the glucose level in blood and also provides sufficient nutrients. As I will discuss later on, if you get used to chewing slowly, you can gradually solve the problem of overeating. Before World War II, it was a common practice in Japan to serve a meal consisting of rice, soup, vegetables, and pickles. It may have been humble, but our ancestors had plentiful energy from such a diet. It may not be necessary to adopt the Japanese diet of those days, but when you consider there was hardly anyone in Japan suffering from diabetes back then, you will come to see that the problem of our increasing rates of metabolic disorder lies in the diet of the present day. Also, there are people who recommend a carbohydrate-free diet, claiming carbohydrates are the cause for weight gain. I believe eating such a diet risks your health in exchange for a temporary weight loss. Carbohydrates *per se* are neither fattening nor unhealthy. The problem is with *refined* carbohydrates, from which much of the life power has been stripped.

Despite all these problems with white rice and white flour foods, the number of people who include brown rice and other whole grains in their diet is relatively small, mostly because of preconceived ideas such as that it tastes worse than white rice and white bread, it is hard to digest and causes stomachaches. Also some feel it is too cumbersome to cook. But easy ways to cook brown rice are now widely available. Even in the United States, you can now find rice cookers with a brown rice mode. You can set a timer on the rice cooker, leave home for work and enjoy steaming rice for dinner when you get back. Also, in order to make it more interesting to the palate, several varieties of grains mentioned earlier; pressed barley, amaranth, ancient rice or beans such as soybeans, red beans, kidney beans, black beans plus a little natural sea salt which is full of minerals may be added. When the rice has cooled down, one can prepare rice balls for lunch and one can prepare rice porridge from leftovers.

When you try brown rice you will feel much more satisfied after a meal than when you eat white rice. This is because the nutrients in the rice are completely different. Once you get used to brown rice, you will know something is missing when you eat white rice, even if you feel full. Of course, even when well prepared, brown rice does have a firmer texture than white rice. The same is true of whole grain bread. Food with texture, however, is better from a health point of view. Foods that are soft and pleasant to taste are popular, but eating them leads to a habit of swallowing soft food without properly chewing. Not chewing enough is one of the contributing factors to lifestyle-related diseases such as diabetes. Once you start cooking and eating brown rice, I suggest that you get used to chewing 30-50 times for each bite. This recommendation to chew food well is not limited to brown rice; I recommend eating slowly and chewing all food well. By chewing well, the bones and muscles of jaws become well developed helping the circulation of blood, which in turn activates brain cells. Also, a salivary gland hormone called parotin is secreted to help rejuvenate the body and prevent aging. There are many other benefits from chewing well, such as improved alignment of teeth, mental stability, and increased concentration. Those people who stay away from whole grains saying they are too hard to eat are giving up these benefits.

Bread made of unrefined whole grains rather than refined wheat will be digested slowly, curbing the elevation of glucose after a meal. The same applies to noodles and pasta, i.e., whole grain pasta or brown rice noodle rather than noodles and pasta made from refined wheat flour. Also noodles made from buckwheat grain have germ and cotyledon inside the grain that are milled together. This is one of whole foods with high nutritional value. Select grains organically grown without pesticides.

I have talked about rice and other grains quite extensively. Now, I will touch on the remaining 35% of the 85% plant-based foods, mostly vegetables, legumes, fruits, sea vegetables, and nuts.

PHYTOCHEMICALS — *COLORFUL VEG & FR.*

Trace nutrients such as vitamins and minerals are found in abundance in vegetables and fruits. Recently, phytochemicals are getting attention as the seventh nutrient. Phytochemicals are the chemicals for pigment, aroma, and bitter taste. Unlike the five nutrients (carbohydrates, protein, fat, vitamins and minerals), they have no direct relationship to metabolism and therefore have not been regarded as nutrients. Recent research, however, shows that phytochemicals have an antioxidant effect suppressing the spread of cancer cells and repairing damaged cells. It is expected that they can also boost immunity from infectious diseases as well as boost memory and concentration. Of the 10,000 phytochemicals existing in nature, the most well known are polyphenols. Anthocyanin, which is the pigment composition of grapes and blueberries, isoflavone in soybeans, and catechin which is the bitter taste in polyphenol foods, carotene found in carrots and pumpkins, lycopene in tomatoes, lutein found in corn, broccoli and spinach are known as phytochemicals of the polysaccharide group. Fucoidan which is sticky and found in sea vegetables, glucan in fungi, pectin in apples and grapefruits are all phytochemicals.

These phytochemicals have been created by plants for their own survival in nature. For example, when a plant is exposed to strong ultraviolet rays, a large amount of active oxygen, which is a free radical, is generated, damaging cells and preventing the growth of the plant. Polyphenol and carotenoid exercise their antioxidative effect to render such ultraviolet rays harmless. Another example is the bitter or sharp taste or the unpleasant odor of plants so that insects or small animals will not eat them, a function of phytochemicals.

Fresh vegetables and fruits are packed with enzymes and robust life power. By eating fresh vegetables and fruits, we are receiving their life power to nourish our own. You can therefore understand why it is necessary to examine the quality of each food in order to make sure you are getting plenty of phytochemicals, vitamins, minerals and enzymes from the vegetables and fruits you eat. The important point is to select produce that is fresh and organically grown in fertile soil. Eating vegetables and fruits is very important, but choose carefully. The way they are grown is key to their nutritional value.

Animal source food should represent no more than 15% of our diet, with 85% of our diet coming from plant sources. Animal source foods may be divided into fish, meat, eggs, milk and milk products. The biggest problem with these foods is that excessive consumption will result in the degeneration of our intestinal features, which is linked by my observation to various diseases.

The fats in fish and meat are different, although both are animal source foods. Unsaturated fatty acid called omega 3 in fish such as EPA (eicosapentaenoic acid), DHA (docosahexaenoic acid) is known to lower cholesterol levels, but you should not take it in excess. Large fish such as tuna or swordfish more and more often these days are tainted with mercury. Mercury stored in a human body can cause severe damage to the nervous system. It is, in fact, known that mercury stored in the body of the present population is on the rise. Better to refrain from excessive eating, even of fish.

As a rough guideline, I recommend a daily consumption of 100g or so of seafood, usually in the form of small fish such as sardines or pompano fish, which have less risk from mercury contamination, or boiled-dried baby sardines which are rich in calcium. Meat tends to make blood dirty and deteriorate intestinal features so it is best to have good quality beef only once or twice a month in a small serving. I advise chewing meat very well both to savor the taste and to promote digestion. Eating fritters or deep-fried foods may cause indigestion and may result in excessive intake of trans-fatty acid. It is more advisable to sauté lightly in cold pressed oil such as extra virgin olive oil or good quality sesame seed oil, or to cook without using oil by grilling or stewing.

With regard to eggs, it is all right to have fertilized eggs from free ranging hens one to three times a week. It is better to avoid milk and milk products (butter, cheese, yogurt, cream, etc.), which can cause problems for many people.

Protein is broken down into amino acids in the body and is an important substance as the base of 40–60 trillion cells. Out of approximately 20 amino acids that make up protein, nine are referred to as essential amino acids and they cannot be synthesized within the body. In other words, unless they are supplied from daily meals, it is possible to develop deficiencies causing problems to health and overall life functions. The reason animal source protein is called high-quality protein is because it contains all nine essential amino acids. However, no matter how ideal the composition of protein may be, this does not mean that all of the amino acids can be absorbed in the body. Also meat, milk and milk products, typical animal source proteins, are all high in fat content and calorie content, and have little dietary fiber. One should moderate the eating of these foods and refrain from making them a large part of one's

brown rice + beans = essential amino

diet. Consider eating traditional, humble meals based on beans, brown rice, greens and a pickle for digestion. This ordinary cuisine is more or less universally recognized. In the American south it is "hoppin' john" or black-eyed peas and rice, in the Carribean it is black beans and rice, in Mexico it is brown beans and rice, and in Japan it is brown rice with soybean soup or natto. Neither rice nor legumes have sufficient essential amino acids by themselves, but, when combined, they supplement each other to give you the nine essential amino acids. When miscellaneous grains, vegetables, and fungi are added to the above, there will be more amino acid supplemented. Combining foods correctly will provide an adequate amount of amino acids without the problems connected to eating animal protein. Of course, over-consumption is never recommended, even when the food is plant-based, but these combinations of simple dishes can provide amino acid protein without a burden on your health. I think it is clear that animal-source protein is not necessarily required to sustain life.

key

The core of the Shinya diet, which consists of plant-source foods, may seem dull to people who are used to eating meat. However, I would like you to think about how the glut of these meat-heavy meals is exhausting your body and mind. It is entirely possible for red-blooded Americans to cultivate a taste for meals based on plant source foods, and life will feel much better in the healthier body you have as a result.

Of course the major premise is to select the best quality foods possible, which means food with life power. Should you feel a lack of strength after adopting a diet-and-health method of mostly plant source food, it is possible that the vegetables or fruits you have selected have lost life power from pesticides or chemical fertilizers, or, in the case of processed foods, from various additives in them. If it is difficult to get fresh foods with energy, it may become necessary to take supplements such as vitamins, minerals, or enzymes.

Even if you are able to get fresh, organic food, it will be difficult to prepare a tasty and healthy meal if ingredients for cooking such as salt, and oil are of poor quality. Most of the salt sold in our supermarkets is refined salt, which is produced from sea water by artificially extracting sodium chloride. It may look like salt, but it is quite different from natural sea salt, which contains other minerals such as magnesium, calcium, potassium, and iodine. Food manufacturers have learned to extract the main component, sodium chloride, leaving out all the other minerals in the seawater and then call it salt. Such a refined salt is like a man-made chemical substance, and its excess intake will result in an imbalance inside the body causing hypertension and other problems. If you are using an appropriate amount of natural sea salt rich in minerals, there is no need to worry about hypertension and it should not be necessary to reduce salt intake.

White sugar is produced by a refining process that loses most vitamins and minerals, leaving only a sweet flavor and calories. White sugar is quickly absorbed by the body, and thus its excessive intake will result in a rapid increase of glucose in the blood, causing diabetes and obesity. In addition, sugar is an acidic food and therefore its intake in large volume will distort the pH balance of the blood resulting in excessive acidity. Our body maintains its balance in a mildly alkaline state, so to neutralize excessive acidity, the body must release minerals to restore alkalinity. The one mineral consumed most by the body for this task is calcium.

The majority of our body's calcium is found in our bones. When a large amount of calcium is wasted, our bones get weaker and could become porous as in osteoporosis. Trace amounts of calcium are also needed in our cells and blood, so a deficiency of calcium distorts the balance of mind and body causing irritability, anxiousness and lack of concentration. The increase in the number of people who lose their temper at trivial matters could be attributable to a large intake of white sugar, depleting calcium. We consume too much white sugar by eating pastries and cakes and drinking soft drinks. If you must have something sweet, try unrefined dark sugar, natural maple syrup, or pure honey without additives. The natural way to get carbohydrates for use as an energy source for the body is to get them from unrefined grains (brown rice, whole wheat foods) or unrefined sugars, which will not cause a sudden elevation of the glucose level.

Condiments such as miso paste or soy sauce with reduced sodium tend to include extra additives. Also there are quite a few miso paste and soy sauce products that are miso and soy in name only. You should be careful in your selection and try to choose products that are naturally brewed utilizing natural fermentation. Fermented foods benefit us because in the fermentation process microorganisms break down protein to amino acids facilitating its absorption by the body. Also, further enzymes are activated, increasing the constituents of vitamins and minerals that can be absorbed.

LIFE POWER IS PROPORTIONAL TO THE AMOUNT OF ENZYMES

I have tried to explain the function of nutrients such as carbohydrates, vitamins, and minerals in your body. Now I want to take you further into understanding your health and explain the very important function of enzymes, which are indispensable for all our life activities.

I wrote an entire book about enzymes, called *The Enzyme Factor.* Briefly, enzymes are protein-type substances involved as catalysts in all phases of life activities. The pumping of our hearts, breathing, digesting, absorbing and eliminating food, thinking, and even feeling are all functions dependent on enzymes. For plants germinating, growing, spreading leaves, blooming, bearing fruits and nurturing new life would not be possible without enzymes. There are 3,000 to 5,000 known enzymes, but probably this is just a fraction of the enzymes in our body. Unless these enzymes are functioning properly, all the nutrients from even the most balanced diet cannot be utilized. We wouldn't be able to sustain our life activities even for a moment without enzymes.

Generally enzymes are categorized into digestive enzymes, which are involved in digestion and absorption of food, and metabolic enzymes, which convert the nutrients to various energies necessary for life. There are certain amounts of enzymes stored in our body, but they can become depleted by poor dietary habits which impair intestinal features, drinking alcohol in excess, smoking, stress, drugs, toxic substances in our environment, electromagnetic waves, ultraviolet rays and so forth. When you eat a diet of meat, milk, and milk products, more enzymes are required to aid digestion. If you work all day at a desk using a computer and talking on a cell phone, you will be exposed to electromagnetic toxins, and enzymes will be required to destroy the free radical oxygen generated inside the body. If you continue a lifestyle that depletes enzymes you will exhaust your body's ability to digest and metabolize food, and your cells will lose their ability to repair themselves. As a result, your life power will decline.

The more we use up our enzymes through a destructive lifestyle, the less life power we will have, leading to disease and death. When a person is lively and vibrant with life power the enzymes within his or her body are fully functioning. If enzymes are depleted, it is difficult for a person to be really healthy no matter how excellent medical care may be. The lack of understanding of the role of enzymes in our bodies and the control they exert on our health has led modern medicine to a system of symptomatic therapy where patients are treated for symptoms.

What is needed is a way to activate the enzymes to invigorate our minds and bodies, and this means we avoid a lifestyle that consumes enzymes. In addition to an enzyme-rich diet, good quality water, moderate exercise, and a calm, stress-free mind are important. Food enzymes are easily destroyed by heat and therefore raw vegetables, fruits, fish, and fermented foods are the best sources for food enzymes. By aggressively adopting an enzyme-rich diet, which focuses on these foods, one can make up for the depletion of enzymes.

AN ENZYME IS BOTH A SUBSTANCE AND NOT A SUBSTANCE

Enzymes are catalysts involved with the core elements of life activities. There are many aspects of enzymes that our science and research have only begun to uncover, and there are many areas where we have to rely on hypothesis. For example, enzymes are considered to be made of protein. It has been pointed out that when you supplement enzymes through food you eat, the food will be broken down to peptide and amino acids and therefore you have not really supplemented enzymes. It is true that enzymes are made of protein, but this does not mean they are the same as protein. I have been using an expression "protein-type substances." Some researchers in the U.S. use the analogy that the protein is the vehicle and the enzyme is the driver. Unless there is an enzyme as driver, a protein vehicle will not move.

Today, many people live mostly on junk food, convenience food, fast food, food heated by microwave ovens, canned foods, and frozen foods. We have little opportunity to eat vegetables and fruits freshly picked and loaded with enzymes. Even when we can eat raw vegetables and fruits, the vitamins and minerals contained in these foods may have little life power because the soil in which they were grown has been deteriorated with the overuse of pesticides and chemical fertilizers. In other words, the life-power-source, enzymes, contained in the foods most of us eat has been reduced.

This is the reality, and yet if we follow the guidelines of the present-day nutritional science which consists of caloric calculation and analysis of nutritional components, all foods are analyzed on the same basis whether they are junk foods, prepared by a microwave oven, vegetables cultivated in exhausted soil or fresh vegetables grown in fertile soil. I believe the most important calculation — how much life power is in the food — has been ignored. Visualize the refreshing sensation when you bite into a fresh tomato grown organically in fertile soil. Don't you think it is a strange nutritional science that breaks down all foods to their respective components then analyzes them for respective nutrients? Once we understand the nature of enzymes, which are the source of life power, we have to make a fundamental shift in our thinking about the food we eat and the earth that produces that food.

ORIGINAL MODEL FOR ALL ENZYMES

There are many aspects about the work of enzymes we have not yet learned. Each type of enzyme can perform only one function. For example, an enzyme called amylase, which is found in saliva, works to digest carbohydrates, and an enzyme called pepsin found in the stomach works to digest protein. Each one is for one specific purpose and thus there are several thousands to several tens of thousands of enzymes. I cannot help thinking that maintaining so many different enzymes is a suspiciously inefficient system for our very efficient human body. I think there must be one basic source, a prototype enzyme, a "miracle enzyme" as discussed in *The Enzyme Factor,* from which the body can create all those other types of enzymes as needed.

When one consumes excessive amounts of alcohol, a large number of enzymes are required to break down the alcohol in the liver. When the enzymes needed to break down the alcohol are generated, enzymes for digestion and absorption in the stomach become scarce. On a day after heavy drinking people often lose their appetite. The lack of available digestive enzymes could explain such a phenomenon. Although individual enzymes can work on specific functions, you can see that they are not functioning independently but are coordinating with each other.

A person who cannot drink much alcohol at first gains the ability to drink more as he gets more used to drinking. This implies that the number of enzymes available to break down alcohol in the liver is increasing by responding to the need. This phenomenon is not limited to alcohol consumption. SOD (super oxide dismutase), which eliminates free radicals in the body, can increase its secretion if you eat more anti-oxidative foods such as fresh vegetables and fruits.

It is based on these fact patterns that I have formed the hypothesis of the miracle enzyme. My theory is that enzymes taken from food are not only being broken down to amino acids but are also pooled as prototype enzymes in the body, and that these prototype enzymes are then transformed into the thousands or tens of thousands of enzymes that respond to the various activities and needs of the body. I think that various individual enzymes morph from this prototype enzyme.

Living a lifestyle that strains the supply of the prototype enzyme, or miracle enzyme, will cause one to develop functional deficiencies throughout the body diminishing one's life power. In order to increase life power, it is important to efficiently supplement enzymes through our daily diet. The "natural" way to do this is to eat meals consisting of fresh raw vegetables and fruits, which have an abundance of enzymes. If my theory is correct, these food enzymes will be stored as miracle enzymes, the source for all kinds of other enzymes in the body. By activating our body's enzymes with the right food, we can attain mental and physical health and improve life power.

LET'S EAT MORE RAW FOOD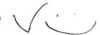

Current medical and nutritional science doesn't have a very developed understanding of the work of enzymes involved in the core of life activities. It may be more accurate to say that our current medical and nutritional science has a lack of interest in enzymes. Thus, prevailing theories of health care are far apart from the realities of our daily life.

In modern medicine, it is expected to use anticancer drugs for cancer treatments. As you may know, when anticancer drugs are used, often patients will suffer from severe side effects such as nausea, loss of appetite, loss of hair, and diarrhea. The reason for such severe side effects is that these anticancer drugs are deadly poisons, which will damage not only cancer cells but also normal cells. When normal cells are damaged by these deadly poisons, a large number of enzymes are necessary to repair these damaged cells. Thus the enzymes that have been pooled by the body as miracle enzymes are depleted, causing a deficiency of enzymes throughout the body. A deficiency of enzymes will lead to a poor physical condition with severe side effects.

Such damage is not limited to anticancer drugs. All drugs inhibit the activities of enzymes. We should realize that it is poisoning one's own life power to readily use drugs in order to suppress a symptom. By taking a cold medicine you may get relief from some of the symptoms of the cold, but your immune power will gradually become weaker and you will be prone to diseases. I myself am fully aware of the problems posed by drugs and try to avoid using drugs as much as possible. For example, even when an operation is necessary for a cancer, I seldom administer anticancer drugs after cancer cells are removed. Instead, I instruct patients to change their lifestyle.

In particular I recommend the adoption of Shinya Biozyme, which I explain in this chapter. The food we eat on a daily basis makes up the cells in our bodies. A good diet that enables the supplementation of our miracle enzyme will improve our intestinal features and lead to steady recovery after an operation. Of course, in order to lead a life free from cancer and other diseases, it is better to start practicing the Shinya Biozyme when one is in good health.

Think of chimpanzees in the wild, many of whom live out their natural life span. What is the basis for such good health? One cause may be the raw foods wild chimpanzees consume. Daily consumption of raw plants results in replenishing enzymes, which are the source of life power. Literally, by supplementing life from foods, one is nourishing one's life.

We need to stop eating dead foods without enzymes. I apologize for being repetitious, but this is an important issue given little attention by traditional nutritional or medical science in today's United States. Could we be healthy by eating calories and nutrients as recommended by the food pyramid? If that is the case, then why do we have a health and obesity crisis in America? I think it is good to reflect on this issue.

Chapter 8

Gain Vitality from Plant Power

VEGETABLES AND FRUITS ARE FOODS
FOR STAMINA AND AN ACTIVE LIFE

Plant-based foods such as vegetables, fruits, and sea vegetables are a rich source of nutrients. When you eat fruits and vegetables you receive the power of life from the plants. Because plant-based foods contain dietary fiber, people who consume sufficient amounts of plant foods have clean-looking intestinal features and have a better balance of good bacteria while there is hardly any garbage buildup in the colon producing toxic waste. I have observed these results through my forty years of experience performing endoscopic examinations of more than 350,000 people. A mere observation of stool makes it clear. The stool of people who consume abundant plant-based food doesn't have a bad smell, is soft and tends to float in water. It is my belief that a diet rich in plant foods has more power to nourish human life and bring out the health of body and mind than a diet primarily of animal-based foods. Plant-based foods will support your life force so that you can lead an active, vital life into old age. Essentially, health is based on the condition of our intestines, and that condition improves with a diet based 80% on plants.

PLANT-BASED FOODS HELP SUPPLY THE BODY WITH WATER

One of the reasons I recommend eating fresh vegetables and fruits is that these plant-based foods are 70–90% water. Eating plant-based foods will help the body get good quality water. In addition to drinking plenty of fresh water, I urge you to consume fresh fruit or fresh juice of vegetables and fruits. Throughout a day, it is better to snack on fresh fruit in season, rather than eating cookies and candies. Consumption of fruit is a part of the Little Fast I mentioned earlier. When eaten 30-40 minutes before a regular meal, fruit will help prevent excessive intake of carbohydrates. Fruits after meals, however, should be avoided because eating them then will have an opposite effect leading to an excessive intake of carbohydrates.

WATER IS AN IMPORTANT NUTRIENT

Most of us don't drink enough water. Our cells are 80% water, and I believe almost any physical problem can be improved by drinking enough good water.

We cannot sustain our life without water no matter how many other nutrients we get in good proportion. It is said that we eliminate about 2.5 liters (10.5 cups) of water every day as urine and sweat. Unless our bodies are rinsed in such a way, the sanitary condition inside us deteriorates and hazardous substances generated in our intestines will oxidize all the body's fluids. Edema, constipation and various other diseases result from a lack of water. In order to prevent such a situation it is necessary to drink plenty of good water. Supplying good water will help to flush out dirty water and improve the circulation of body fluids. Good water becomes good body fluid flushing and eliminating dirty fluid from our cells.

WHAT IS GOOD WATER?

Now that we know that it is important to supplement with water, what kind of water should we be drinking? Much tap water contains large amounts of chlorine used for sterilization as well as other hazardous substances called trihalomethanes, which are carcinogens generated during the sterilization process. Also, tap water may be contaminated by agricultural pesticides and fertilizers, industrial pollutant runoff, and other wastewater treatment residue that makes its way into aquifers, reservoirs and groundwater supplies. Water is tested, of course, but even though these substances may be within the scope of government safety standards, this is hardly the proper water to nourish the cells of the entire body.

Depending on where you live, you may find it desirable to install a water purifier to remove chlorine and hazardous substances so that you can drink water closer to its natural healthy state. Thirty years ago in Japan we were worried about the amount of acid rain we were getting in our water. A group of scientists, engineers, and doctors including myself got together to talk about what we could do to save our water. Out of that meeting a technique was developed to process water in order to make it more alkaline. Others went on to build a machine that does this, for people to put in their homes. I am a doctor and that is my work, so I didn't get involved in any of the business, but since that time I have been drinking this alkaline water we call Kangen water. The technology for producing the Kangen water has gotten much more sophisticated, of course, and Kangen water machines have become available in the United States. I have a Kangen water machine in my New York medical office, and this is the water I drink and give to my patients. In addition to filtering out pollutants this Kangen water has strong reduction power and helps keep the body at an optimal alkaline pH.

Generally an adult man or woman loses 2.5 liters of water as urine and sweat every day, and therefore there would be a deficiency of water in the system unless one takes in at least the amount of water lost. If you assume the water contained in foods is 1 liter, we need to supply the body with a minimum of 1.5 liters (6.5 cups) of water. When it is hot in summer or on the days of increased exercise, more water will be needed. We should try to drink eight cups of water so we have a little cushion. If you are unable to drink so much water it could mean you are chronically deficient in water. The cells which make up our body, blood and lymph fluid are metabolized by the water you take in, so that drinking more water will help you to maintain fresh and youthful skin and make your cells active. Of course it is important that the water be of the quality I have just outlined.

THE BODY DOES NOT WANT TEA, SPORTS DRINKS OR ALCOHOL

In supplementing water do not include beverages such as tea, soft drinks, coffee, and alcohol as part of your water intake. It is not a good idea to skip water and quench your thirst after sports activity by drinking sports drinks. Although many of these drinks have minerals and amino acids necessary for the body, they may also contain a large amount of sugar. When all this sugar is consumed, your glucose level surges and a large amount of insulin is secreted from the pancreas. This is a burden on the body and the body will feel sluggish and tired afterward.

Teas have a healthier image than high-sugar soft drinks, but when the stomachs of people who drink tea every day are examined through an endoscope, their mucous membranes often look rough. I believe this is caused by tannin, a bitter substance in tea. From ancient times, there have been high numbers of people who have stomach ulcers or stomach cancers in cultures where tea drinking is a regular feature, such as among the Japanese. Moreover, tea contains larger amounts of caffeine than coffee. Caffeine has a strong diuretic effect, so that most of the water in the tea you drink will go right through you and be excreted without hydrating your cells. In other words, you may be drinking tea thinking you are slaking a thirst, but you are actually dehydrating yourself on the cellular level.

It is also a bad idea to gulp down chilled beer when you are thirsty. You may feel immediately good with the increased circulation from the effect of the alcohol, but after a few hours your blood vessels will shrink making it difficult to supply oxygen and nutrients to cells. It will also burden the body by compromising the elimination of waste.

Like tea, alcohol is highly diuretic and will dehydrate, not supplement, water to the body. Beer after playing sports will not resolve the water deficiency caused by sweating. You may have exercised for health and accelerated metabolism, but if your exercise ends with a beer or two afterward, it will actually contribute to the aging of your cells.

It is important to minimize soft drinks, sports drinks, energy drinks, alcohol, and tea as mentioned above and not to equate drinking those kinds of liquids with drinking water. Water is what your cells want. Drink a cup or two of water at regular intervals during the day. In this way, you retain the moisture content of your cells thereby protecting yourself from cellular degeneration and disease.

BOTTLED OR CANNED FRUIT JUICE
MAY BE DEVOID OF ENZYMES

Even though vegetables and fruits are good for your body, you should not substitute bottled or canned fruit juice for water. When you see a label claiming 100% fruit juice, look to see if it also says it is made from concentrate. Enzymes in Group A are lost through the process of applying heat to create concentrated juice. It's best to eat fruits whole or juice them yourself. Vegetables may be consumed as juice, salad, or fermented products like kimchi or pickles. By thinking of the life force of your food you will see why freshness is necessary and why organic plant foods grown in good soil without chemical fertilizers are best.

TEA AND COFFEE ARE NOT WATER

There is another reason why I do not recommend drinking coffee, tea or soft drinks in the place of water. With regard to coffee and tea, it is harmful to consume excess caffeine. Also coffee drinks on the market often contain refined sugar and milk. Catechin in tea is claimed to be good for health, but my observation through endoscopic examination suggests its excess consumption might lead to stomach cancers. Many carbonated drinks in my opinion are polluted water saturated with sugar. These sugary drinks will induce elevated blood sugar levels, which can lead to diabetes. You may think when you are consuming these liquids that you are satisfying your body's need for liquids, but these drinks will not bring the benefit of good water. One simple change you can make in your lifestyle that will improve your health is to make good water your beverage of choice in situations where you have been drinking beer, coffee, tea, sports drinks, or sodas.

ENZYMES ARE INDISPENSABLE FOR ALL LIFE ACTIVITIES

Enzymes are indispensable for our life activities and function as intermediaries for all chemical reactions in the body. They are called catalysts and without them there could be no chemical reactions. Enzymes are needed to breakdown the nutrients of foods in the stomach. Enzymes to break down protein are different from enzymes to break down carbohydrates. For each reaction, a specific enzyme is required, and enzymes are not interchangeable. There are 3,000 – 5,000 types of enzymes in the human body, perhaps more. Since our life is composed of numerous chemical reactions, it can be said that enzymes are the source of life. Needless to say, specific enzymes are involved in intracellular detoxification. There are some 60 varieties of enzymes involved in the detoxification work of proteolysis, or autophagy. I call these enzymes newzymes or rejuvenating enzymes. When these rejuvenating enzymes are functioning properly, cells are healthy with a fresh moisture content. If there were no enzymes we would not be able to sustain our life even for a second, since enzymes are involved in digestion and absorption, breakdown of toxins, breathing, moving, heart function, and brain activities.

Rejuvenating enzymes

Enzymes are the source of life and are indispensable for our life activities. They are also found in plants. For example 90% of plant cells are sack-like organs containing vacuoles. These sacks contain not only water but also numerous detoxification enzymes. These enzymes that have the ability of detoxification are classified as rejuvenating enzymes— newzymes. Fresh vegetables and fruits look juicy because of water in their vacuoles, but this water would quickly fill up with garbage (waste and hazardous substances) if left alone. Newzymes inside vacuoles, however, take care of such garbage thus maintaining the freshness of fruits and vegetables. It is also the work of rejuvenating enzymes to ripen and sweeten fruits. Such fruits as pineapples, kiwi fruits, papayas and figs have newzymes with very powerful ability to decompose cellular garbage. When you have a cold or feel tired, you feel refreshed when you eat fruits. This is because you are replenishing enzymes in your body. You are getting vitamins and minerals as well, but these are nutrients to support enzymes and cannot function by themselves. It is necessary for them to have synergetic interactions with enzymes.

Consume raw foods

The more cooked food you consume, the more difficult it is to supply enzymes. Even if you are getting vitamins and minerals from such food you will not be deriving the benefit of enzymes. The labels on fast food or processed foods may say they contain the same amount of nutrients as fresh raw food, but the enzymes and the life force will not be the same.

How to select an enzyme supplement

Depending on the way enzyme supplements are produced, their effects on the body fluctuate widely. The definition of an enzyme supplement has not been clearly established and you may be surprised to learn that there are products on the market labeled enzyme supplements which don't even contain enzymes.

Enzyme supplements should be produced using natural vegetables and fruits, which are then fermented with microorganisms. Enzymes are not resistant to heat and if during the process of production they are heated to a temperature of 48°C (119 ° F) or more, their function is reduced to nothing. Only the non-functional enzymes remain in the finished product.

In the U.S. most enzymes on the market are digestive enzyme supplements such as protease (enzyme to break down protein), amylase (enzyme to break down carbohydrate), and lipase (enzyme to break down fat). They are typically produced using a low temperature or no heat so that the enzymes will not be destroyed.

The Japanese have been using enzymes for centuries for many health benefits and cultivating enzymes through the fermentation process is an art. Master vintners carefully cultivate special microorganisms for many years to make sure it is the strongest and the best culture. This culture is then used to activate the fermentation process of naturally grown vegetables and fruits. Enzymes produced in such a way are functional enzymes and are not treated with any heat. The best enzyme supplements are processed to maintain a trace amount of water in the enzyme powder in order to maintain the enzymes' life force in a state of suspension until they awaken when taken into the body. This type of enzyme has the added advantage of supplying effective microorganisms. I have been interested in the cultivation of enzymes for many years and have helped develop a special enzyme I call ShinZyme. This enzyme is not a digestive enzyme but a support for intercellular detoxification and the immune system.

MINERAL DEFICIENCY –
CRISES OF OUR PRESENT-DAY LIFESTYLE

Let's go over the function of vitamins and minerals in Group B. These nutrients supplement the function of enzymes and thus they are often referred to as coenzymes. Enzymes have a leading role in life activities, and minerals and vitamins, which are coenzymes, coordinate with enzymes to facilitate the smooth function of respective organs and body systems.

Minerals are sodium, magnesium, phosphorous, calcium, chromium, manganese, iron, copper, zinc, selenium, molybdenum, iodine and so forth. The amounts of these minerals in our body are very small, but when we are deficient, the function of enzymes will deteriorate, impairing life activities. When you are feeling slack, tired, unmotivated; when you catch cold easily, lose control of your emotions easily, or are irritable or depressed, a deficiency of minerals may be involved. Such symptoms are ubiquitous in our world today.

There are more than 100 varieties of minerals and they are classified into (1) major minerals, and (2) trace minerals. Among major minerals, the best known mineral is calcium. Among minerals, the amount of calcium requirement for our body is the highest. Calcium makes up our bones. Additionally approximately 1% of the calcium in our body helps in the functioning of our blood, nerves and muscles. This 1% of calcium has a very important role in maintaining the health of our body and mind. Functions such as clotting of blood, stabilizing nerves, promoting hormone secretion, and facilitating smooth movement of muscles are dependent on this calcium. When there is not enough calcium in our diet for such important functions, the body will supply this calcium by taking it out of our bones. If such a situation becomes chronic the calcium in our bones will become depleted and osteoporosis can be the result. When this 1% calcium is deficient we can feel on-edge, become frustrated easily, and even lose emotional control.

Minerals cannot be produced in the body, and thus we must supply them through foods. Each mineral has a distinctive function in our body's life activities and its shortage will have an adverse effect on our health. Trace minerals such as iron, zinc, copper, iodine, and selenium are much smaller in their volume when compared to major minerals such as calcium, magnesium and potassium, but this does not mean that major minerals are more important than trace minerals. Each of the trace minerals has its own role and functions by teaming up with others. It is important to supply *all* of them.

HOW TO GET THE MINERALS YOU NEED

Animal-based foods contain minerals but are hard on the health of the intestines. I recommend plant-based foods such as vegetables, fruits, sea vegetables and natural, unrefined salt. But there is a problem. Much of today's agricultural practice uses chemical fertilizers instead of rich, composted soil; therefore soil's traditional treasure house of natural minerals is not available in most produce. Chemical fertilizers are composed mainly of nitrogen, phosphoric acid and potassium. These minerals are good for the growth of plants, but when they are the major components of nourishment, the balance of minerals is compromised. In other words, the life power of plants has been reduced. You can imagine that the life power of the people who eat these plants has declined as well. One solution is to support sustainable agriculture by eating vegetables and fruits that are cultivated in organic soil, which has a good balance of minerals. Minerals are not destroyed with heat, and we can eat vegetables as soup, stew and so forth. We can also make enzyme juice from fresh carrots, cabbage, spinach, parsley and other colorful vegetables.

MINERAL SUPPLEMENTS

If you are concerned about getting enough minerals from your food you might consider taking a good quality mineral supplement.

Some say that supplements are not natural and one should refrain from a complete dependence on them, but since natural produce may not have adequate minerals or enzyme power, it is wise to make careful use of supplements.

I recommend taking supplements with natural ingredients especially those extracted from plants, rather than those which are synthetically produced. It is important not to take one ingredient excessively such as calcium only or iron only. In this sense, it is a good idea to take multi-mineral supplements.

VITAMINS

Vitamins are similar to minerals in that they coordinate life activities. Different from minerals, they are organic consisting of numbers of elements. Over 20 vitamins, such as A, B group (B_1, B_2, B_6, B_{12}, etc.), C, D, E and so forth have been identified, and each has its unique function. The function I want to discuss is vitamins' action as an antioxidant, removing "rust" and rejuvenating the body. This antioxidant action is found mostly in vitamins C, E and the B group. The rust of a body is called oxidation — in other words, aging. As aging, or oxidation, progresses, the skin, veins, organs and brains all lose their youthful vitality. Vitamins are necessary ingredients in anti-aging.

What is oxidation? A part of the oxygen breathed into our bodies is changed to radical oxygen while it is being converted to energy inside our cells. On the most elemental level, the O_2 molecule loses an electron. These electrons, or free radicals, are the cause of oxidation. Protein inside a cell is damaged by radical oxygen and becomes deficient protein or garbage. Radical oxygen may be generated from stress factors or electromagnetic rays from computers, cell phones, ultraviolet rays, smoking and other environmental factors.

Ordinarily, radical oxygen is made harmless by specific enzymes, but when the load of oxidized "garbage" protein becomes too great, the work of enzymes may not be enough. Some may argue aging is natural, but the process of oxidization of cells by radical oxygen is accelerated in the presence of many unnatural environmental factors today.

PHYTOCHEMICALS

Antioxidant functions are not limited to vitamins. Phytochemicals in Group C have similar functions. Phytochemicals are unique elements supporting the life of a plant. You may have heard of catechin and isoflavone. They are members of polyphenol, which is one of the phytochemicals. Beta carotene and lutein are in the carotenoid group of phytochemnicals. Aroma, bitterness, and color are important chemical strategies for plants. For example, excessive exposure to ultraviolet rays causes free radicals to be generated thus damaging cells in plants and humans alike. The phytochemical polyphenol minimizes such damage. Bitter taste and special scents are the work of phytochemicals protecting plants against insects and animals. Phytochemicals are part of a plant's life power. I believe we have only begun to understand the importance of phytochemicals for human health and nutrition. Phytochemicals may be called assistants to minerals and vitamins, which are coordinators.

85% PLANT-BASED FOOD AND 15% ANIMAL-BASED FOOD

My opinion as a physician who has been observing intestinal features for many years, is that an ideal diet consists of 85% plant-based food and 15% animal-based food.

To make my advice very simple, practice the Shinya Fast by drinking enzyme juice in the morning. Drink eight cups per day of good water and eat fresh fruits and vegetables with legumes and brown rice or other whole grains. Add a small portion of fish once or twice a week, preferably a small fish, like sardines, which do not have too much mercury.

- A diet of vegetables and fruits gives you stamina

- Water is an indispensable nutrient for life

- You cannot get enzymes from fast food

- You cannot get minerals and vitamins from a diet of white rice and meat

BROWN RICE, THE PERFECT FOOD

My first recommendation for protein in your diet is brown rice with soybeans. Through this diet, one can get sufficient amount of essential amino acids. If you add other types of legumes or grains, you will be getting even more protein. If you add small fish such as sardines, or sea vegetables, you will be getting enough protein without relying on meat. Brown rice with soybeans and other grains with plenty of dietary fiber will lead to smooth evacuation and detoxification of the intestines. Food does not have to be digested promptly. It is better if digestion takes a little time. Japanese who have dieted on foods with rich dietary fibers are known for relatively long intestines. It is important to question how smoothly foods are absorbed rather than concerning oneself with the types of nutrients.

FISH

Fish, like meat, contains good quality essential amino acid. Additionally it has good quality fat, which is not found in meat. You may have heard of EPA (eicosapentaenoic acid) or DHA (docosahexaenoic acid). These are found in fish and are called unsaturated fat or omega 3, and they cleanse blood and decrease the serum triglyceride level. One of the problems with eating meat is that animal fat thickens blood. Fish is a much healthier source of food. Through my experience, I have confirmed that people who eat fish have much better intestinal features than those who eat meat. Diverticulitis is seldom found in people who eat fish. Feces and toxic substances tend to accumulate in a diverticulum and if nothing is done about it, it can lead to colon polyps or cancers. There is a problem, however, with eating fish, and that is the contamination of seawater from which the fish are taken. Large fish, such as tuna, contain high levels of mercury and excess consumption of tuna may lead to troubles of the nervous system. In marine life, small fish are eaten by medium size fish, and medium fish are eaten by large fish, and thus large fish have the highest concentration of mercury.

SMALL FISH AND SOYBEANS ARE
A TREASURE HOUSE OF COLLAGEN

There are foods that are rich sources for the amino acid that is the material for collagen. The benefit of collagen is not limited to the health of skin. Collagen makes up bones, joints, muscles, tendons, blood vessels and other bodily tissues. Calcium is known as the material for bones. If you compare a bone to a building, calcium is like a concrete wall. Without collagen, which might be compared to the iron frames of a building, there would be no bone. Ligaments and tendons are mostly made of collagen. The epidermis of the skin and the inside wall of vessels are also made of collagen. Thirty percent of all the protein that makes up the human body is collagen. Small fish is recommended as the source of collagen because of the high quality collagen, which is found in the scales of the fish. Some say that collagen is a kind of protein and therefore it is broken down into amino acid and will not remain as collagen. However, it is not essential amino acid and therefore it can be synthesized inside the body. As much as 30% of our body is made up of protein, and therefore I recommend supplementing collagen. One of the reasons I recommend soybeans is they contain amino acids such as glycine and proline, which are the major components of collagen. Collagen supplements extracted from scales of fish are available on the market, but it might be better to get this valuable nutrient from small fish and soybeans.

- Excess intake of protein deteriorates intestinal features (health barometer of intestines)
- Brown rice with soybeans is the recommended source of protein
- Small fish and soybeans are a source for collagen, a necessary element for beautiful skin

Chapter 9

Healthy Intestines Lead to Healthy Cells

Since healthy intestines are so essential to human health, I focus many of my recommendations on lifestyle practices that keep them clean and functioning well.

Many people suffer from chronic constipation. Those who have not improved their dietary habits inevitably have trouble with bowel movements. Some don't have a bowel movement for several days, while others have hard stool, running stool, or irregular volume of stools.

It is not necessarily OK just to have a bowel movement on a daily basis. The following points should be checked.

1. Hardness of stool. It should not be too hard or too soft. (A banana-shaped stool is ideal.)

2. Amount of stool. The volume of the stool should relate to the volume of food consumed on the previous day. If it is too little, you have constipation.

3. Odor of stool. If a foul smell is present, it is a sign that your intestinal features are in a bad state. If you feel gassy after a bowel movement, it means you have feces remaining in the upper portion of the large intestine.

4. If you feel a sense of incomplete evacuation, you have constipation.

A healthy evacuation is free from those four points and the feces has little odor and has a shape of a banana. It varies depending on your physical condition and you need not be too nervous, but if you fail in the above checkpoints, you have constipation. It does not necessarily lead to sickness immediately, but with such a physical condition, you cannot expect efficient detoxification of cells. Constipation will most likely lead to chronic fatigue, and a sense of weariness or frustration. Constipation is caused by your daily diet.

COFFEE ENEMA TO CLEANSE INTESTINES

For those people who have constipation or who are suffering from swelling of extremities, an intestinal cleansing may be in order. One means to cleanse the colon is a coffee enema, which I have been recommending to my patients for many years.

The coffee enema is an intestinal cleaning method established by a German physician, Max Gerson, in 1920, to evacuate feces stuck in the lower portion of a large intestine. It takes only 15 minutes or so, including the preparation time.

- Add water to coffee solution in a container to make a three-cup solution at body temperature.

- Hang the container on a wall in a bathroom and insert a hose attached to the container into the anus for an inch or so.

- Release a clip attached to a hose to let coffee solution enter the intestine.

- When the container is empty, evacuate.

The coffee solution is made from organic coffee beans and is free from chemicals which may cause diarrhea. It will not remain inside the intestine after evacuation. Feces stuck in the intestine will be evacuated and you will feel relieved. You will not become addicted to it. This will eliminate the constipation that is the cause of your discomfort.

Generally glycerin is used for an enema to induce peristaltic motion of an intestine and it should not be used too frequently, because such use will impair the natural intestinal functions and make you dependent on it. Those people who now depend on laxatives may adopt a coffee enema so that they will increase good intestinal bacteria while restoring peristaltic movement.

COFFEE ENEMA HELPS LIVER FUNCTION

Why is coffee used for an enema? In 1920 when the use of a coffee enema was developed, O. A. Mayor and Martin Hubner, two doctors of Gottingun University in Germany, researched and confirmed that caffeine in coffee expands the bile duct for a smoother flow of bile to help the function of the liver. The liver is the largest organ in our body and it breaks down toxic substances generated by garbage in our intestines. Drinking coffee will not result in such an improvement. The quality of the coffee used is important. Instant coffee sold in the market will not work. In order to maximize the benefit, it is important to use coffee solution made from high quality organic coffee. Dr. Max Gerson (1881-1959) pioneered the use of the coffee enema in his alternative treatment for cancer. After it was confirmed in 1980 that an active constituent in coffee supports the breakdown of toxins in blood, more health practitioners began to incorporate the coffee enema into their practice.

METHOD TO CLEAN COLONS

For my patients and myself I have developed an enhanced coffee enema. It has been 80 years since Dr. Gerson developed the coffee enema, and our environment and dietary habits have changed. There are increasing numbers of foods to taint our intestines. For forty years I have been observing through my endoscope the effect our increasingly toxic diet has on our intestines. That is why I have created the Shinya coffee enema which adds lactic acid bacterium, oligosaccharide, to facilitate the cleaning of colons, as well as enzymes and sea salt rich in minerals. The Shinya style coffee enema uses only the highest quality organic coffee. Of course it is also critical to use good water for the solution. You may use mineral water commercially available although it is necessary to bring the temperature to the body temperature.

There are clinics that offer colon-cleaning services using machines, but I don't recommend this because machine-fed water may elevate the pressure inside colon and could possibly damage the bowel wall or aggravate diverticular inflammation. Also, they cleanse the colon repeatedly, and there is a danger that minerals in the colon may be flushed out.

I am not saying that you can gain health by just cleaning your colon. The coffee enema is a safe, efficient means to eliminate impaction caused by the consumption of toxic foods.

USE OF HERBS FOR A BUSY LIFE

While I was studying various herbs, I noticed that the petals of flowers contain substances which are effective for cleaning intestines. To be more specific, flower buds, right before blooming when the life force is at a peak, are most effective. The combination of the coffee enema with these herbs will enhance the cleansing of the intestines. Peach flowers are known for their effect on puffiness, constipation and menstrual pains; orange flowers promote the functions of intestines; Japanese honeysuckle has a diuretic effect and helps peristaltic movement of intestines; Tibetan safflower reduces sensitivity to cold and helps with menopause problems; a type of carrot lowers cholesterol and triglyceride, and adjusts the autonomic nerve system. These buds are the treasure houses of phytochemicals. Chinese medicines are known for a combination of various herbs to maximize their effect, but the problem here is their taste. I combined them with coffee in a drink. The taste of coffee neutralizes the bitter taste of these herbs. One can take them on a daily basis or one can substitute this for the coffee enema when busy.

MASSAGING – EXCELLENT MEANS FOR DETOXIFICATION

I have covered morning fasting, coffee enemas and herbs (buds of flowers combined with coffee). In order to facilitate the cleansing of intestines, it is helpful to have several options and to combine them effectively, as indicated by the condition of your body. As one more option, I would like to introduce massaging of the intestines. The method was devised by Yasue Isazawa, an aroma therapist, and I will call it the IM method (intestinal massaging method). It takes only 5-10 minutes. It has a very positive effect and is easy to perform.

WARMING UP:

1. Lie flat on your back and relax.
2. Breathe in from the nose and expand the abdomen
3. Breathe out from mouth and flatten the abdomen
4. Repeat the above 10 times

KNEADING OF LARGE INTESTINE:

1. Bring the knees up and bring both legs to the right side
2. Knead your abdomen on the left side (the lower part of large intestine where stool tends to accumulate) 10 times, slowly with your left hand
3. Repeat 3-4 sets of 10

KNEADING OF SMALL INTESTINE:

1. Place fingers (thumb, index finger and middle finger) of both hands at about an inch above the navel and slowly knead in a clockwise rotation 10 times
2. Slide the fingers down and repeat the kneading around the navel.
3. Repeat 3 sets. Concentrate in the area where you feel pain.

It is easy to practice. You can combine taking herbs followed by kneading or work on kneading followed by coffee enema and so forth.

A CHANGE IN DIET CAN HELP RELIEVE DEPRESSION

People suffering from depression often take anti-depressant drugs or sleeping pills. The intestines of people who take that kind of medication are often black from the precipitation of pigments. In addition those with depression often have constipation or diarrhea. When we don't have a good diet, good rest and good elimination we will naturally suffer from emotional and mental distress. Remember the expression, we are what we eat. In other words the contents of what we eat will determine the quality of our cells, and those cells will make up our intestines, brain, muscles, nerves and organs. Food that is bad for your intestines cannot be good for your cells, your brain, or your nerves. I think it makes sense to start the treatment of depression by considering the state of your intestines. When you feel frustrated, uneasy, or depressed, I advise you to first check your diet and bowel movement. It is better to improve your diet and cleanse the garbage from your intestines and cells than resort to medications.

GUT IMMUNITY

Immunity refers to the body's defense mechanism against bacteria and foreign elements that try to invade the body. It is our resistance to disease. One of our most powerful defense functions is in our intestines. About 60–70% of our immune cells are concentrated in the Peyer's patches cells in our small intestines. The small intestine is an organ whose role it is to absorb nutrients from the food we eat. Nutrients are absorbed by numerous prongs called villus which fill the inside walls of the small intestine. There are countless numbers of spaces in villus where immune cells are clustered, and they are called the Peyer's patches. In other words, if an intestine is not clean, the function of these immune cells (generally referred to as gut immunity) will be compromised and this will compromise the resistance of the whole body. In order to elevate our immune power, it is necessary to follow a diet which will not contaminate our intestines and to employ detoxification methods such as the Shinya fast. Most diseases can be prevented without resorting to medications by maintaining clean intestines.

- Cleansing of intestines is indispensable for the health of cells
- Breakfast fasting with water and fruits (the Little Fast) is the easiest detoxification method
- Shinya-style coffee enema is recommended for bad constipation or puffiness
- Simple kneading of intestines leads to activating immunity

DEEP BREATHING INVIGORATES CELLS

We absorb oxygen by breathing through the lungs and then sending the oxygen to all the cells in the body through our blood vessels. Nutrients in food are also carried to our cells where they are changed to energy (ATP) by mitochondria, but no matter how many nutrients are present no energy can be generated in the cells unless there is an adequate supply of oxygen. You may think that would never be a problem since we are always breathing. The level of our cell metabolism varies, however, depending on how we breathe.

Find a comfortable place to sit. Breath normally for a few moments, then:

- Breathe in through your nose making a balloon of your abdomen with your breath
- Hold for a few seconds
- Breathe out slowly taking about five seconds feeling yourself relax as you do so.
- Repeat for five or six breaths

Zen practitioners practice a similar breathing technique. It promotes rejuvenation of mind and body by sending abundant oxygen to the cells. By taking in more oxygen, one can effectively utilize nutrients without building up garbage in the cells. By stimulating the diaphragm located between lung and intestines, the peristaltic activity of the intestines is enhanced. When frustrated or angry our breathing becomes shallow. Because of this not enough oxygen gets to our cells and our metabolism is compromised creating problems with digestion and absorption. Breath deeply always and, when possible, take a few minutes to practice abdominal breathing. Deep breathing elevates your innate immune power.

Mouth-breathing triggers contagious infection

An important point to keep in mind is to practice nose-breathing rather than mouth-breathing. There is a difference. Our nostrils are covered with countless hairs and mucosa. These are filters to prevent the invasion of viruses, bacteria, and dust. We breathe in air and send it to the lungs after filtering it through the nose. The cells that make up the mucosa have numerous sensors to catch foreign elements.

Cancer

Having cancer does not have to be solely a negative experience; it gives one a chance to review one's way of life, and to make a change to a healthier lifestyle in order to prevent its recurrence.

The primary focus of my work is to show how disease can be prevented. I would much rather help prevent cancer, for example, than try to cure it. Still there are many cases where people are already ill and there are increasing numbers of people who have developed cancer. Of course it is best to prevent cancer but if you are already facing a cancer diagnosis, what should you do? Surgery, chemotherapy and radiation are still the three major treatments prescribed by physicians. Even with these measures, however, there is sometimes metastasis and recurrence. When cancerous cells are removed, there is no guarantee that they will not recur. Treatments of chemotherapy and radiation have side effects such as loss of hair, inflammation of skin, vomiting, and an extreme sense of exhaustion. Some cancers such as colon cancers or breast cancers have high survival rates if detected and at early stages. Early detection and treatment are not a complete solution, however, and one may remain prone to reoccurrence.

There are treatments, however, in the field of alternative medicine, to support the remission of cancers. One noteworthy treatment is an intravenous administration of high-density vitamin C. This method was established by twice Nobel Prize winner Linus Pauling. In the beginning, the method was not widely accepted, but in 2005 the National Institution of Health delivered a report in support of it. According to Pauling's thesis, vitamin C administered intravenously will turn to hydrogen peroxide, which attacks cancer cells. Hydrogen peroxide is a kind of free radical and is harmless to normal cells, so that, unlike radiation and chemo, it doesn't poison the body. Dr. Pauling established the Molecule Nutrition Study and is known as one of the pioneers advocating natural medicines, which are not dependent on chemicals.

EVERGREEN TREE WITH POWERFUL ANTICANCER EFFECT

The interesting point of the vitamin C intravenous therapy mentioned above is that vitamin C when infused in large volume turns into a free radical. It may sound shocking, but free radicals by themselves are not harmful and function as a part of our immune mechanism. When the number of free radicals increases excessively, then they become harmful. Vitamin C which has turned into a free radical (hydrogen peroxide) will attack only cancer cells. A nutrient which is necessary for the health of our body becomes our defender attacking rogue cells. There is ongoing research with other substances besides vitamin C to find allies in our effort to weaken or terminate cancer cells. Among these substances are numerous phytochemicals. One that intrigues me is produced by an evergreen tree from the Yunnan province of China. Many domestic organizations are studying its powerful anti-cancer properties. Similar to concentrated vitamin C, it selects and attacks cancer cells specifically. Furthermore, it can induce cancer cells to their apoptosis. Due to apoptosis, cancer cells cannot split any further and will become the prey of phagocytes such as macrophages. A substance prouced by this tree also has the ability to inform macrophages that cancer cells are not ordinary cells but are foreign elements. Macrophages specialize in devouring foreign invaders such as viruses or bacteria but when fed with the extract of this tree they will recognize cancer cells as foreign invaders even though the cells once were normal. These natural anti-cancer substances also have properties that can improve our body's anti-aging functions or strengthen our innate immune power.

Chapter 10

Practical Guide to Elevate Your Innate Immune Power

THREE POINTS TO ELEVATE INNATE IMMUNE POWER

In order to rejuvenate cells and lead a healthy life of mind and body the following three methods are recommended.

I. THE SHINYA LITTLE FAST.

The foundation to elevate innate immune power is to induce intracellular detoxification through fasting. I recommend the Shinya Little Fast. Here is how you do it:

1. Finish dinner by no later than 7 P.M. (ideally by 6 P.M.).

2. Upon awakening drink 2–3 cups water.

3. Instead of breakfast, have some fruits. An enzyme juice of apples, cabbage, carrot juice, etc., is also recommended.

4. Drink 2–3 cups of water before lunch.

It is important not to consume any heated or cooked food in morning hours. Drink water before dinner also. A daily consumption of 6-8 cups of water is recommended.

Learn to enjoy the sense of feeling hungry. Feeling hunger is an indication of intracellular detoxification.

II. INTESTINAL DETOXIFICATION.

Practice intestinal detoxification for further effect. Detoxification of waste, garbage and hazardous substances inside intestines will lead to intracellular detoxification to vitalize the functions of cells. The following three methods are recommended:

1. Coffee enema or coffee enema with flower buds.
2. Flower bud coffee drink. There are coffee flower bud capsules for busy people.
3. Massage intestines 5 to 10 minutes per day.

III. SHINYA STYLE DIETARY HEALTH METHOD.

In addition to fasting and intestinal detoxification, a staple diet of whole grains and legumes is recommended.

Eat 85% plant source foods and 15% animal source foods. Reduce the consumption of meat and increase the consumption of vegetables (including rice) and fruits to 85% of your intake.

Eat fermented foods and fungi. Fermented soybeans, pickled vegetables and fungi will elevate immune power.

In addition to the above three points, try to practice deep breathing through the nose. Also get in touch with nature: hiking, farming, gardening, etc., to elevate your innate immune power.

Remember that most of our immune power begins in our intestines, and our health is based on the vitality of cells.

Practice these three points to build a body that will fend off diseases.

Chapter 11

Shinya Beauty Plan and Your Natural Weight

Vibrant good health is beautiful. The beauty regimen I recommend includes the Shinya Biozyme, which I have already described. If you diligently practice the diet and health method I am advocating, you will not need any other special diet for shaping-up. This is because your everyday meals will be continually rejuvenating your cells and making your intestinal features clean. Your skin will become smoother and firmer, and you will naturally return to a healthy weight.

Those people who want to make an improvement in a short time without stress on the body should follow these 3 rules.

1. Drink 1.5–2 liters (6–8 cups) of good water every day
2. Have smooth bowel movements one to three times per day
3. Aggressively include living foods in the daily diet for a steady supply of enzymes

Simply stated, the three keys to the Shinya Beauty Regimen are:

1. good water
2. natural elimination
3. food enzymes

WATER

The first essential is water. Water is the most important aspect of the Shinya Biozyme. The reason why water is the first essential is because drinking an ample amount of good water is an easy health and beauty regimen, which almost anyone can practice. I don't think the importance of water as an aid to health and beauty has been fully acknowledged. Of the many beauty regimens and diet methods, few list good water as the key essential. The idea that one can get healthy or look younger just by drinking water may seem too simple to be true. In order to understand why this is so, it will be necessary to explain the importance of water.

It goes without saying that water is indispensable for maintaining our life and that 60–70% of our body is water. Where is the water stored? The answer is obvious, if you think what constitutes our body. It is stored in our cells. There are an astounding 60 trillion cells making up our body and these cells are mostly water. Besides the water in our cells, our intracellular fluid, there is water flowing in our circulatory organs, namely blood and lymphatic fluids. These are referred to as extracellular fluids. Both our cells and our circulatory organs are metabolized daily with water where waste products and toxins are broken down and excreted. Excreting waste and toxins is the most important essential to a successful health and beauty diet and regimen.

Generally an adult man or woman loses 2.5 liters (10.5 cups) of water as urine and sweat every day, and therefore there will be a deficiency of water in the system unless one takes in at least the amount of water lost. If you assume the water contained in foods is four cups, we need to supply the body with a minimum of six cups of water. When it is hot in the summer or on the days of increased exercise, more water will be needed. We should try to drink six to eight cups of water so we have a little cushion. If you are unable to drink such an amount of water it could mean you are chronically deficient in water. The cells which make up our body, blood and lymph fluid are metabolized by the water we take in. We must drink more water in order to maintain fresh and youthful skin and make cells active. Of course it must be good water. I urge people to understand the meaning of good water, which I am going to explain, and to put that knowledge into practice.

Now that we know that it is important to supplement water, and not just any beverage, what kind of water should we be drinking? Much tap water contains large amounts of chlorine used for sterilization as well as other hazardous substances called trihalomethanes, which are carcinogens generated during the sterilization process. These substances may be within the scope of government safety standards, but it is hardly the proper water to nourish the cells of the entire body.

Depending on where you live, you may find it necessary to install a water purifier to remove chlorine and hazardous substances so that you can drink water closer to its natural healthful state. Some water purifiers are designed not only to remove toxic substances but also to release natural minerals by installing carbon or mineral ores inside a cartridge. Natural water contains rich amounts of minerals from soil and rock as it travels from its source through groundwater veins to the surface of the earth. By switching your habit from drinking tea, coffee, carbonated beverages, and so forth, to good water, your physical condition will improve.

With regard to the amount of water to drink, I recommend 1.5 to 2 liters (6–8 cups) per day. I myself drink 500–750 milliliters (2 or 3 cups) each morning, afternoon and evening. Basically I drink water immediately after I get up, and an hour before lunch and dinner. Additionally, you should drink frequently, adjusting to the weather, amount of exercise, body condition and so forth. As a reminder, try not to drink ice-cold water. The same applies to other beverages or ice cream, because cold intake will lower your body temperature and lower cell activities. The consequence will be a lowered immunity and a body constitution prone to diseases. Drink water at room temperature. Take time to drink it, and when you feel it has reached your intestines, eat some fruits. I will explain later why I suggest fruits at this time.

How to remove garbage in the intestines

After you get used to drinking good water, I want you to become aware of what I call natural bowel movements. Many who have a bowel movement every day may still be troubled with hard stools or small volume excretion. This problem is generally not taken seriously, but constipation is one of the leading causes of impaired intestinal features.

Some physicians don't regard constipation as a disorder unless it causes severe symptoms. This is because many don't fully understand what is happening inside the intestines when stools accumulate.

The stools accumulated in an intestine are, simply put, like garbage. If you leave garbage out in heaps in summer it will decay and develop a foul odor. The same is true inside the intestine. Hazardous substances such as hydrogen sulfide, phenol, skatole, indole, ammonia, methane are generated, and the intestines fill with strong-smelling gas. As a consequence, there will be the propagation of bad bacteria and further deteriorating intestinal features. Free radical oxygen will also be generated. These hazardous substances will be absorbed into the bloodstream and carried to cells throughout the body. In this manner, when intestinal features deteriorate, body fluid becomes tainted and cells themselves are damaged.

This is why, when constipation persists, one will develop rough skin and lose the firmness or glow of the skin. The toxins generated from the garbage inside the intestines will have adverse effects on cells throughout the body. Also the interruption of the flow of oxygen in the blood can cause chronic fatigue, stiff shoulders, backaches, headaches, and menstrual cramps.

If intestinal features deteriorate from the effects of constipation, there is an increased risk for the onset of diseases of the colon, such as colon polyps, colon cancers, and ulcerative colitis or Crohn's disease. On the other hand, a clean colon will result in the rejuvenation of cells as the foundation of beauty and health. Eliminating waste and toxic substances inside the body is generally described as detoxification. Sweating in exercise or in a steam bath or sauna is helpful, but it is far more effective for the purpose of detoxification to improve bowel movements. Quite a few people claim they feel all right when they don't have good bowel movement for a few days, but they should realize that by accumulating garbage in their intestines, they are depriving themselves of their youth and in some instances they are shortening their lifespan. Good elimination is even more important to health than good nutrition.

METHODS FOR NATURAL BOWEL MOVEMENTS

Following a diet such as the Shinya Biozyme is the first step toward improving bowel movements. The most important practice in the diet is minimizing the intake of animal source foods (meat, milk and milk products), which are bad for digestion, and instead to include unrefined grain which is rich in dietary fibers, and vegetables, including sea vegetables. Specifically brown rice, sea vegetables such as kelp and agar, and root vegetables such as yams are recommended. If you prepare a Japanese style meal of rice, miso paste soup, and boiled food, the intake of dietary fibers will be plenty. The intake of dietary fibers will be significantly reduced with a meal containing lots of meat and fat. It is also important to eat large amounts of raw foods rich with food enzymes. These foods include fresh fruits, raw vegetables, and fermented foods. These foods contribute to the generation of enzymes in the body, good bowel movement, and stable intestinal features.

If you are beginning this diet for the first time, you may get started by simply switching your staple food to brown rice. If you combine such a diet with a sufficient quantity of good water, your intestinal features will improve and your bowel movements will improve as well. It may be easy to say to improve your eating habits, but it is possible that you may not be able to improve your diet as much as you would like. For those who work outside the home, it may be necessary to dine out during the day. Remember, chewing well and eating slowly are very important. Even if you try to be careful about where you eat and what you order, often you may end up in a hurry, eating fatty meat without chewing enough. In this way, you may fail in the regimen, even though you know it is a good method. In such a situation I would suggest a coffee enema, which can improve intestinal features in a short period of time. I have been administering coffee enemas to myself for more than 30 years. I am over 70 years old and I believe the coffee enema, along with my diet, has kept me actively working as a physician in two countries flying back and forth between New York and Tokyo. Also I have more elastic skin than many much younger people.

LIVING FOOD (RAW FOOD)

I have been explaining about Shinya style beauty regimen and diet method with the key words of good water and proper elimination. Now, I will talk about supplementing food enzymes, which is the other essential. Raw vegetables and fruits are rich with enzymes, which are the source of life energy. Many people are turning their attention to meals and diet methods using raw food, which is full of enzymes — living food. The raw food movement was developed in United States, which is the best place for enzyme nutritional science.

An easy way to put living food into your diet will be to eat enough fruits in the morning hours, to drink juice of fresh vegetables and fruits prepared using a blender, to eat fresh salad before meals and chew them well. These are all efficient ways to supplement enzymes. I recommend eating fruits in season if possible. I recommend drinking good water one hour before breakfast, lunch and dinner, followed by eating fruits 30 minutes before meals. In this manner, the intestinal work is energized, resulting in smooth bowel movement If you have some carbohydrates (fructose) before a meal, overeating can be discouraged.

Fruits after a meal will lead to an excess intake of carbohydrates causing weight gain. Therefore I don't recommend this. It is better to eat fruit frequently during the day. Those who are concerned about overeating can switch from snacks such as pastries or cakes to fruits. Switching from pastries and cookies loaded with white sugar and milk products to dry fruits and so forth will lead to an improvement of the body's constitution. Many people in the U.S. are obese from the excessive intake of animal source foods, fast foods, transfats, and so forth. If you are overweight or obese, you can benefit by simply increasing your intake of raw fruits or vegetables. This will improve your intestinal features and lead to a more natural diet. Smoother circulation of blood will improve the skin and lessen allergic symptoms.

Many vegetables and fruits found in our markets have much lower life power than those produced in the past. The amount of vitamins and minerals in these foods has been drastically reduced when compared with the same food produced 50 years ago. This implies that the life power of produce has come down as well. When the amounts of vitamins, minerals, and coenzymes (cofactors to help the work of enzymes), have been reduced, it is unlikely that the essential enzymes can be working actively. If the enzymes are not adequately functioning, the life power of produce must be lower also. Perhaps that is why the raw food diet (raw vegetables and fruits) alone seems not to be enough to elevate the life power. I am aware of the importance of supplementing living food and enzymes, and that is why I mention the raw food approach developed in the U.S. with respect, even though I perceive the limitations of a strictly raw food diet.

SUPPLEMENT ENZYMES AND COENZYMES

What can we do to deal with the shortage of energy or diminished life power of the vegetables and fruits available to us? I think we should focus on taking good quality supplements. By supplementing vitamins and minerals and enzymes, which might no longer be found in vegetables and fruits, not only will we be able to improve our health, but also we will be able to increase our life energy. Take enzyme supplements to help digestive enzymes in the body, and multi vitamins and multi minerals containing necessary trace components in a good balance before and/or after meals.

People who are working full-time tend to have irregular meals. By adopting the Shinya Biozyme, by incorporating the coffee enema as needed, and by taking good quality supplements, even those working hard and unable to eat as regularly and carefully as they wish can have good health and feel less tired. As metabolism is invigorated, one can expect good results in rejuvenating the tone of the skin. The vitamins our body requires are vitamins A, B_1, B_2, B_6, B_{12}, C, D, E, and K. As for minerals, calcium, magnesium, phosphorus, iron, zinc and selenium are some examples. These vitamins and minerals are required in a small amount when compared to the amount required of the three nutrients — carbohydrates, protein and fat; however, vitamins and minerals are components which support the functions of enzymes (coenzymes) and therefore when they are in a short supply our life functions such as digestion, absorption, metabolism and excretion are compromised. Also, one becomes prone to irritability, unstable emotions, and listlessness. Having a shortage of the life power in the vegetables and fruits we eat every day, we have become a people suffering from chronic deficiency in vitamins and minerals.

With regard to the types of supplements you should look for, basically choose those extracted from natural components, rather than those synthetically produced. Regarded from the viewpoint of elevating one's life power, the natural product would be preferable.

MACROBIOTICS

A macrobiotics diet is an "alternative" health method that became popular after World War II. In Japan, Yukikazu Sakurazawa based his ideas about macrobiotics on the work of Sagen Ishizuka, a physician in the Meiji era. Triggered by the references to a traditional Japanese diet mentioned in the McGovern report, macrobiotics rapidly became popular in the U.S. during the period from 1980 through 1990. Ironically, now that Americans are adopting this healthful Japanese tradition, the Japanese are imitating the Americans and there is a macrobiotics boom in Japan.

The basis of the macrobiotic diet is a staple of brown rice, various cereals, unrefined whole grain wheat flour in combination with supplementary dishes of vegetables, legumes, and sea vegetables, avoiding animal source foods such as meat, milk, milk products, eggs, or fish. The macrobiotic diet promotes eating local produce, based on the concept that our body and the environment are inseparable, as well as eating whole foods based on the concept of taking in the whole life power in the food. All foods are grouped into yin, yang, and middle path, and depending on the body type of an individual a combination of foods from respective groups are chosen to achieve a balance. This balance between yin and yang is considered essential in macrobiotics. In principle, it is a diet and health method that focuses on the relationship between food and people, a practice of eating and living according to the natural order, thereby achieving the health of mind and body. It is understandable that it is accepted in the U.S. and Japan as a reaction against agribusiness and the western-style diet.

The difference in the Shinya Biozyme and the macrobiotic method is the Biozyme's emphasis on enzymes and life power. Many macrobiotic recipes recommend that living foods be prepared by stewing or sautéing. This means vital enzymes are destroyed in the preparation of everyday foods. Also I am concerned that too many macrobiotic recipes use fat. Some sautéing is all right, but deep-fried foods such as croquettes often found in macrobiotic lunches have an adverse effect on intestinal features. Even if good quality foods are used, they are not recommended as necessary to the macrobiotic diet. Further, there is a not enough about the importance of drinking good water and proper elimination. There are many concepts I admire within the macrobiotic diet, such as the concept regarding food as life, but I don't think it goes far enough in its understanding and therefore should not be accepted as-is.

I have compared both the raw food diet and the macrobiotics diet with the Shinya-Biozyme I am advocating, but it is not my intention to emphasize the differences. In a broad sense, they are all classified as natural diet methods with an emphasis on the connection between foods and body. These diets are all full of helpful suggestions one can incorporate into daily meals.

THE LOW CARBOHYDRATE DIET

On the other hand, there are wrong dietary health methods —beauty regimens and diet methods that have dangerous effects. The common denominator of these methods is, in short, based on the concept of reducing one's carbohydrate intake. The most typical example is the Atkins diet developed by Dr. Robert C. Atkins in the U.S. This diet, in my opinion, is a high-risk diet, which induces oxidation of blood and leads to deterioration of intestinal features. One may be able to temporarily lose weight on such a diet, but there is a high probability of damaging one's health.

In order to understand why the elimination of carbohydrates is dangerous, you will have to understand the function of a hormone called insulin, which is secreted from the pancreas. The carbohydrates we ingest from foods are sent to our bloodstream from our intestines, boosting the glucose density in our blood. It is the function of insulin to lower such glucose levels. If one keeps consuming too much carbohydrate, the pancreas gets tired, impacting the amount of insulin secretion. Diabetes is a disease that develops as a result of this kind of stress on the pancreas. The idea behind low carb diets was to so severely lower the intake of carbohydrates that insulin would not be secreted. Furthermore, it was thought that once there was no carbohydrate for the body to convert to energy, the body would attempt to break down body fat to generate the energy it needed. The concept of this kind of diet is that it would lead to the slimming of the body by burning stored fat. Body fats are stored in a body for an emergency such as famine, and are difficult to break down as the source of energy. The no-carb or low-carb diet intentionally creates a pseudo-emergency by restricting the intake of carbohydrates. Unfortunately in exchange for breaking down stored fat, a substance called ketone is generated which causes the body fluid to become acidic. When the body fluid is acidic, cells deteriorate resulting in functional deterioration of muscles and organs. In some instances, a disease called ketoacidosis caused by the oxidation of the blood may develop.

LOW INSULIN DIET, ONLY A THEORY

There are other problems with diets that restrict carbohydrates, like the Atkins diet. While there is a restriction on the intake of carbohydrates (grains such as rice, bread pasta, etc., pastries with sugar, fruits, legumes, potatoes, etc.), it has no restriction on the amount of animal-source foods (meat, milk and milk products, eggs, fish, etc.). Animal-source foods don't have dietary fiber and contain a high percentage fat and calories, thus there is a risk of developing dense blood and deteriorating intestinal features. Also, due to the insufficient oxygen and nutrient supply to cells throughout the body, energy metabolism is hampered, leading to the aging of cells. You will see that the idea of losing weight by just reducing the intake of carbohydrates, which was conceived by only considering the issue of insulin, resulted in a nearsighted concept without any regard to the organic connections of the entire body.

For thousands of years the Japanese have had a diet of abundant carbohydrates mostly from unrefined grains, with a minimum amount of animal-source foods. This is exactly the *opposite* of low carbohydrate diets. There was no adverse effect on the health of the Japanese. In fact, obesity and diabetes hardly existed in Japan prior to World War II. Only after the Japanese adopted the western-style diet and started consuming excessive amounts of animal-source foods did problems such as obesity and metabolic syndrome or insulin resistance become an issue.

As long as one is concerned about losing weight at any cost, disregarding such undeniable facts, one will end up compromising health in exchange for short-lived success.

The same is true with the diet method based on the body's glycemic index. The glycemic index, or GI index, ranks carbohydrates according to their effect on blood glucose levels. According to this diet method, foods with a low GI index require low levels of insulin secretion. The idea is that low GI foods will not cause weight gain even if one consumes such foods in abundance. As mentioned earlier, the concept of deciding what to eat in accordance with the amount of insulin secretion is simple and clear, but at the same time there are many risks involved. Obviously white rice and white bread have higher GI values and elevate the glucose level more than brown rice and miscellaneous cereals, so the GI index is a helpful tool to a point, but if you go by that standard only, you will quickly get into trouble.

For example, animal-source foods such as beef and pork have low GI values. Milk and milk products also have low GI values. We have already discussed the consequences to the intestines of eating those foods in abundance. It is better to aim for a natural diet that will not cause a burden on the body. It may be true that if one consumes foods with low GI values, the elevation of glucose level will be prevented and one may lose weight and body fat. However, there is no consideration in this diet about how food is digested, absorbed, converted to energy and the wastes excreted. If one is aware of the effect of excessive consumption of animal-source food on intestinal features and how that will cause changes to the health of blood and cells, it should be clear that such a diet is not a healthy one. Rather than narrowly focusing on one aspect of metabolism and one narrow goal of weight loss, take the view of improving overall health of mind and body. A diet based on unrefined grains, legumes, raw vegetables and fruits, good water and intestinal detoxification is, I believe, much better for rejuvenating your health and life power. This is the natural diet that is the key to youthful energy and beauty.

THE IDEAL DIET TO PROMOTE HEALTH, BEAUTY AND REJUVENATION

It is most important to eat unrefined whole grains such as brown rice and cereals. As the staple of your diet, they will be the foundation of your health. Do not substitute dead food or white rice from which all the major nutrients have been removed and do not eliminate whole grain as a staple as a way to lose weight. As mentioned in this chapter, you should not be mislead by one-sided and biased nutritional arguments and should judge by understanding the basics and following the natural order.

Start the day with deep breathing and simple exercise followed by slowly drinking 500-700 milliliters (two to three cups) of good water. After about 20 minutes when the water reaches the intestines, eat seasonal fruits to supplement enzymes, vitamins, minerals and carbohydrates. Thirty to forty minutes after later, eat a simple breakfast. My breakfast is nothing complicated and usually consists of cooked vegetables, natto and *nori* (dried seaweed). It takes about two hours for such a leisurely morning, from getting up to leaving for my clinic. I recommend this for anyone who can take this time in the morning as it starts the day in a healthy way and lowers stress while increasing energy for work. For those who are concerned about overeating, it will be all right to have an adequate amount of good water and fruits before leaving home. In this way, they will be fasting until lunch hour and there will be the effect of detoxification. It is not all right to rush, drink coffee, and eat nothing before leaving home. That way stresses the body and is definitely not in the spirit of Shinya fasting.

Drink good water frequently. I make time to drink 500-750 milliliters (two to three cups) of water slowly, one hour before lunch and again one hour before supper. When you eat out, you will find many dishes available to you that may be bad for your intestinal features. In this case it would be better to bring a lunch from home of brown rice. You don't have to be fancy with side dishes. Of course, there are occasions you may have to dine out. In such instances, try to avoid greasy meat dishes, choose wisely and aid your digestion by chewing well. On occasions when you feel you have to eat meat, take enzyme supplements before meals for better digestion.

The important thing is not to become nervous about what foods to avoid, but to be conscious of what you eat and its effect on your intestinal features. Pay attention that what you have eaten is digested properly and waste excreted. If you worry too much about the things to avoid and become unable to listen to the voice of the body, then you are missing the point. Those people who don't know what the voice of the body is can try to observe the frequency of bowel movements and the condition of wastes as a start.

BEAUTY ACCELERATORS

In the Shinya style beauty regimen and diet method I have given you the three essentials for health and beauty: water, excretion, and enzymes. After you have mastered these three essentials in your daily habits you might want to go a little further and carefully try the following health and beauty accelerators.

FASTING IS THE FIRST ACCELERATOR

Some people may think that the purpose of fasting is to reduce weight and body fat by refraining from eating, but I have told you that weight loss is not the important result of fasting. The primary objective of the kind of fasting I recommend is to eliminate toxic substances in the body. Many of us overeat and include animal source foods in our diet, straining our digestion. We also eat processed foods full of additives and ingest considerable amounts of hazardous chemical substances we aren't even aware of.

Our digestive system works night and day to transform and absorb these foods while breaking down and eliminating hazardous substances. If you do nothing to help the body, the detoxification process will fall behind. If you were to work nonstop at your job like your organs work at theirs, you would fall behind in a few days and might even be driven to death from exhaustion. Our body is working hard to support our life. Don't you think we should give the digestive system a rest sometime? To your body, time free from eating – fasting – is a break from work. During this resting period, the waste accumulated in your intestines will be naturally processed and body fluids, blood and lymphatic fluid, cleaned, thus your body and mind will be reset to a refreshed state. This is the greatest health result from fasting. From a medical point of view I do not recommend a fast that is a complete refusal of foods, but a modified fast as described below.

In order to maximize the health effect from the Shinya fast, you should be sure to drink lots of good water and take in living enzymes. Good water facilitates the cleanup of body fluids and cells, and enzymes energize the metabolism of the entire body.

The fasting I recommend is not a complete refusal of all food but a simple fast consisting of good water and fresh fruits containing enzymes. Fasting (refraining from eating) does not mean that you don't eat at all. You will need good water, fresh fruits containing enzymes, and supplements.

Recently, this type of modified fasting has been gaining popularity. There are retreats for fasting, and also some people take advantage of the two days of a weekend to fast at home. I believe that modified fasting, while at the same time increasing the supply of enzymes available to the cells, has the possibility to energize life power. I am actively researching this idea right now and hope to be publishing more soon on the Shinya Fast.

COFFEE ENEMA

Coffee enemas can enhance and accelerate the effect of detoxification.

THE IMPORTANCE OF REST

Nap when you feel tired. Napping doesn't take a long time. Sometimes five minutes of rest with eyes closed is all you need. When I am working in the clinic, I make it a habit to rest for 30 minutes after lunch. You may doubt the effect of only five minutes or 30 minutes of napping, but this is a precious resting time for the cells. Easy does it. Don't let yourself get too stressed at work or concentrate so hard you forget to pause for breaks. Breaks are important to reset the state of continuous mental and physical energy and to bring to your work a refreshed mind. Those whose work is desk-bound should avoid being glued to their computer, and should step out regularly to practice deep breathing or to drink good water. Basically, I don't recommend bringing work home. If you work at home I recommend stopping work at a certain time and closing the door of your office. After I finish working in the clinic, I go home to have dinner and spend relaxed hours until I retire. My dinner is Japanese-style, consisting of mainly plant foods. The staple food is brown rice accompanied by soybean soup, salad, steamed vegetables, marinated food and natto. As animal-source food, I sometimes eat grilled or braised fish. I rarely eat meat dishes at home. I may eat good quality meat in a restaurant once or twice a year.

Don't eat anything after dinner so that excess enzymes are not used at night. You may drink a glass of water an hour or so before bedtime. It is better to go to bed with an empty stomach.

Don't consume alcohol or tobacco for relaxation. These may give you temporary relief but, as time passes, vessels shrink making it difficult to distribute nutrition and water to cells throughout the entire body. These substances also inhibit the excretion of waste, and toxins accumulate in cells resulting in the consumption of enzymes involved in metabolism. Even if you consume good water and good food, if enzymes are wasted, you cannot elevate your life power. This is an important point to remember.

Chapter 12

Listen to the Voice of Your Body

CONSCIOUS HABITS TO IMPROVE YOUR LIFE

Many patients visit my clinic every day. In the process of listening to their dietary histories and health problems, examining their stomachs and intestines with endoscopes, and treating their diseases when necessary, I can't help but think about how I could help each person live in his or her body in a better way. The result of how we have lived every day is recorded in our bodies. It may sound severe, but I will say anyway that much of the pain and sickness we experience is the result of ignorance about how to properly care for the body we are given. Too often we don't know how to listen to the voice of our body. If one doesn't understand good food or good water, and lives in such a way as to waste life force and enzymes because one is too busy to pay attention, it is not unexpected that one will fall ill. Such a life accelerates the aging of cells and drains the energy, especially as one gets older. We shouldn't think suffering and sickness are inevitable, or that we must decline physically and mentally as we age. You can change your fate now by making an effort to wake up to your own body's voice. It is not only I, a physician, who wishes you to make the effort to take better care of your body in order to maintain your vitality and health. Your own body wishes it even more keenly than I do.

What does my body want now? Is it pleased? Is it sad? Is it angry? Does it hurt? Please make time to listen to the voice of your body. By listening to it, your life will change. You will have a clearer understanding of what I have talked about in this book, and you will be able to begin practicing its message.

What you eat today will become the makeup of the very cells of your body and brain tomorrow. It will affect what you do and think. When you adopt the Shinya Biozyme and your intestinal features become smooth and clean, there will be changes not only in your overall physical condition but also in your consciousness and your life. I am not exaggerating when I say your whole life will change.

Eating has such a strong effect on every aspect of your life. If the intestines are stable from good food, your body condition improves and your mind will become more stable. You will not feel frustrated or worried or angry and you will notice that you are seeing things more positively. The answers you are seeking are hidden inside, in your intestines. A journey of the mind sounds abstract, but the small universe of the intestines is the very place to begin such a journey. We find hints for living better with each other in the coexistence and harmony of countless microorganisms, enzymes, and minerals created in the small universe of our intestines.

Appendix

Dr. Shinya's 7 Golden Keys for Good Health

(NOTE: The 7 Golden Keys are reprinted from my book *The Enzyme Factor*.)

USE THESE KEYS TO PRESERVE YOUR BODY'S "MIRACLE ENZYME" AND ENJOY A LONG AND HEALTHY LIFE.

1. A GOOD DIET

1. **85–90% Plant-based foods:**

    a. 50% whole grains, brown rice, whole wheat pasta, barley, cereals, whole grain bread & beans including soybeans, kidney beans, garbanzo beans, lentils, pinto beans, pigeon peas, black, white & pink beans

    b. 30% green and yellow vegetables; root vegetables, including potatoes, carrots, yams and beets[and sea vegetables

    c. 5–10% fruits, seeds & nuts

2. **10–15% Animal-based proteins (no more than 3 to 4 oz per day):**

    a. Fish of any type, preferably small fish as larger fish contain mercury

    b. Poultry: chicken, turkey, duck – small amounts only

    c. Beef, lamb, veal, pork – should be limited or avoided

    d. Eggs

    e. Soymilk, soy cheese, rice milk, almond milk.

Foods to add to your diet:

1. Herbal teas

2. Seaweed tablets (kelp)

3. Brewer's yeast (good source of B complex vitamins and minerals)

4. Bee pollen and propolis
5. Enzyme supplements
6. Multivitamin & mineral supplement

Foods & substances to avoid or limit in your diet:

1. Dairy products such as cow's milk, cheese, yogurt, other milk products
2. Japanese green tea, Chinese tea, English tea (limit to 1–2 cups per day)
3. Coffee
4. Sweets and sugar
5. Nicotine
6. Alcohol
7. Chocolate
8. Fat and oils
9. Regular table salt (Use sea salt with trace minerals.)

Additional Dietary Recommendations:

1. Stop eating and drinking 4–5 hours before bedtime.
2. Chew every mouthful 30–50 times.
3. Do not eat between meals except for whole fruit (If hunger keeps you awake a piece of whole fruit may be eaten one hour before bedtime as it digests quickly.)
4. Eat fruits and drink juices 30-60 minutes before meals.
5. Eat whole, unrefined grains and cereals.
6. Eat more food raw or lightly steamed. Heating food over 118° F will damage enzymes.

7. Do not eat oxidized foods. (Fruit, which has turned brown, has begun to oxidize.)
8. Eat fermented foods.
9. Be disciplined with the food you eat. Remember you are what you eat.

2. Good Water

Water is essential for your health. Drink water with strong reduction power that has not been polluted with chemical substances. Drinking "good water" such as mineral water or hard water, which has much calcium and magnesium, keeps your body at an optimal alkaline pH.

- Adults should drink at least 6–10 cups of water every day.
- Drink 1–3 cups of water after waking up in the morning.
- Drink 2–3 cups of water about one hour before each meal.

3. Regular Elimination

- Start a daily habit to remove intestinal pollutants and to clean out your system regularly.
- Do not take laxatives.
- If the bowel is sluggish or to detoxify the liver, consider using a coffee enema. The coffee enema is better for colon detox and for full body detox because it does not release free radicals into the blood stream, as do some dietary detox methods.

4. Moderate Exercise

- Exercise appropriate for your age and physical condition is necessary for good health but excessive exercise can release free radicals and harm your body.
- Some good forms of exercise are walking (2.5 miles), swimming, tennis, bicycling, golf, muscle strengthening, yoga, martial arts and aerobics.

5. ADEQUATE REST

- Go to bed at the same time every night and get 6 to 8 hours of uninterrupted sleep.
- Do not eat or drink 4 or 5 hours before bedtime, If you are hungry or thirsty a small piece of fruit may be eaten one hour before retiring as it will digest quickly.
- Take a short nap of about 30 minutes after lunch.

6. BREATHING AND MEDITATION

- Practice meditation.
- Practice positive thinking.
- Do deep abdominal breathing 4 or 5 times per hour. The exhale should be twice as long as the inhale. This is very important as deep breaths help to rid the body of toxins and free radicals.
- Wear loose clothing that does not restrict your breath.
- Listen to your own body and be good to yourself.

7. JOY AND LOVE

- Joy and love will boost your body's enzyme factor sometimes in miraculous ways.
- Take time every day for an attitude of appreciation.
- Laugh.
- Sing.
- Dance.
- Live passionately and engage your life, your work, and the ones you love with your full heart.

Glossary

Antibiotic — a substance or compound that kills, or inhibits the growth of bacteria.

Autophagy —the process by which pathogens that penetrate cells, escaping the attacks of antibacterial and antivirus substances, are shredded on a molecular level. The pathogens are identified inside the cell, bagged and shredded by enzymes.

ATP (adenosine triphosphate) — a molecule that transports chemical energy within cells for metabolism.

Apoptosis — programmed cell death, or cell suicide.

Bacteria — a large group of unicellular, prokaryote microorganisms.

Effector cell — an activated T cell.

Enzymes — protein substances that are involved as catalysts in all phases of our life activities.

Eukaryotic organism — an organism composed of cells with DNA enclosed within a nucleus.

Fungus — a member of a large group of eukaryotic organisms that includes microorganisms such as yeasts and molds, as well as the more familiar mushrooms.

Innate Immune System — Our evolutionarily oldest immune system the innate immune systems provide immediate defense against infection. The innate immune system operates continually to help us stay disease-free most of the time.

Lactobacillus — a major part of the lactic acid bacteria group that converts lactose and other sugars to lactic acid making its environment acidic, thereby inhibiting the growth of some harmful bacteria.

Lymphokines — produced by T cells to direct the immune system response by signaling between its cells and attracting other immune cells, like macrophages and other lymphocytes, to an infected site to attack the invaders.

Lysosome — an enzyme that acts to break up food in animal cells so it is easier to digest. —(In yeast and plants, the same roles are performed by lytic vacuoles.)

Macrophages — the first white cells to react to invading viruses, whose job it is to literally capture and devour pathogens.

Metabolic syndrome — a combination of medical disorders, perhaps caused by prolonged stress, that increase the risk of developing cardiovascular disease and diabetes.

Microbe —an organism that is microscopic, too small to be seen by the naked human eye.

Mitochondria — sometimes described as "cellular power plants" because they generate most of the cell's supply of adenosine triphosphate (ATP), used as a source of chemical energy.

Neutrophils — white blood cells that devour invading pathogens.

Newzymes — the term Shinya coined for the enzymes that do the work of intracellular detoxification in animals, plants and microorganisms. He chose to call them "newzymes" because they are enzymes that help to renew the cells of living organisms.

Pathogens— infectious organisms. These include bacteria (such as staph), viruses (such as polio), and fungi (such as yeast).

Phytochemicals — chemical compounds such as beta-carotene that occur naturally in plants. The term is generally used to refer to those chemicals that may affect health, but are not yet established as essential nutrients.

Prokaryote — organism composed of cells with DNA not enclosed within a nucleus.

Proteasome — an enzyme that degrades unneeded or damaged proteins by a chemical reaction, called proteolysis, that breaks peptide bonds.

T cell — cells belonging to a group of white blood cells known as lymphocytes and playing a central role in cell-mediated immunity. They have special receptors on their cell surface called T cell receptors (TCR).

Toll-like receptors (TLRs) —a class of proteins that play a key role in the innate immune system. These receptors catch foreign invaders and secrete antibacterial and antivirus substances. This function is not limited to the cell that has been invaded. By the work of the sensor, other neighboring cells are notified of this danger and all these cells emit antibacterial and antivirus substances directed at the pathogens.

Ubiquitin-proteasome system — part of the innate immune system by which the enzyme proteasome marks "defective protein" and targets those proteins to break them down — shred them.

Virus —a small infectious agent that can replicate only inside the cells of other organisms.

Index

A

acid hydrolases 41
acidic 14, 25, 43, 53–54, 100, 144, 157
acquired immunity 37–39, 49–51
ageless living 1
agriculture 29, 32–33, 61, 116
Akio Sato 69
alcohol 102, 104, 110–11, 124, 150, 154
alkaline 14, 100, 109, 155
alkaloids 47
allergies 32, 46, 61, 86
alternative medicine 131
Alzheimer's dementia 46
amaranth 92, 93, 95
amino-acids 98–99, 101, 103, 105, 110
animal-based proteins 153
animal source foods 58, 67–68, 97, 134, 139, 140, 142, 148
antibacterial 40, 157, 159
antibiotic 18, 19, 157
antibodies 11, 17, 22, 37–40, 49–50
anticancer drugs 105–06
antigen-antibody complex 38, 39
antigens 49
antioxidant 55, 59, 96, 117–18
antivirus 157, 159
apoptosis 46–47, 49, 51–53, 132, 157
artificial insemination 68, 69
Atkins diet 144–45
Atkins, Dr. Robert C. 144
ATP (adenosine triphosphate) 42–43, 129, 157–58
attention deficit 90
Attention Deficit Disorder 91
auto-immune 61
autonomic nerve system 126
autophagy 40, 44–46, 56, 77–79, 82, 112, 157
average lifespan 21

B

Bacillus dysentericus 18
bacteria 1, 5, 13, 19–20, 22–25, 27–29, 31–32, 39–41, 45, 48–49, 51–53, 87, 91, 107, 125, 128, 130, 132, 138, 157, 158; beneficial 5, 23–25, 27–28, 107; harmful 23–25, 27, 157; intermediate 23, 24
barley 35, 91–93, 95, 153
BCG (Bacillus Calmette-Guérin) vaccination 20
beans 68, 88, 92, 95, 99, 124, 153; black 92, 95, 99; garbanzo 153; kidney 92, 95, 153; pink 153; red 92, 95; pinto 153; white 153
beauty accelerators 148
bee pollen 154
beriberi 91
black spot 46
blood 6–7, 42, 49, 59, 67, 69, 76–77, 84, 93–94, 96, 98, 100, 109–10, 112, 115, 119–20, 125, 129, 136, 138, 141, 144–46, 148, 155, 158–59
brains 90, 117
bread 33, 64–65, 85–86, 89–91, 93, 94–95, 145–46, 153
breast cancer 66, 70
breathing 156; deep 134, 147, 150; mouth 130
brewer's yeast 153
brown rice 153
bubonic plague (Black Death) 1, 11, 15–16, 22
buckwheat grain 96
butter 69, 98

C

cabbage 33, 116, 133
caffeine 7, 47, 91, 110–11, 125
calcium 66–67, 89, 92, 98, 100, 115–17, 120, 142, 155

metabolic disorder 94
metabolic syndrome 8, 84, 145
metabolism 26, 43, 76, 90, 94, 96, 111, 129–30, 141–42, 145–46, 149–50, 157
microbes 1, 9, 11–13, 16, 19, 22–24, 30, 36–37
microorganisms 5–6, 12–16, 18–20, 23, 25, 30–32, 36, 46, 48, 68, 101, 114, 152, 157–58
milk 24, 58, 64, 65–70, 76, 85, 87, 91, 97–98, 102, 111, 139–40, 143–46, 153–54
milk products 58, 64, 66–67, 69–70, 76, 91, 97–98, 102, 139–40, 143, 145–46, 154
minerals 30–31, 33, 59, 82, 86–87, 89–90, 92, 95–97, 99–101, 103, 110, 113, 115–19, 126, 137, 141–42, 147, 152–54; deficiency 115; supplements 117
miscarriages 58
miso 24–25, 27, 101, 139
mitochondria 42, 44–46, 48, 75, 78, 93, 129; defective 44
Molecule Nutrition Study 131
molybdenum 115
Montezuma's Revenge 22

N

nap 156
natto 25, 99, 147, 150
nerves 46, 67, 90, 115, 128
nervous system 98, 120
neuronal system 91
neutrophils 25, 37, 39, 50, 158
newzymes 7, 48–49, 52–60, 71, 77, 112–13, 158
nicotine 154
Noboru Mizushima, Prof. 77
NPK fertilizers 29
nucleic acid 54

nutrients 7, 25–26, 31, 33, 41–45, 51, 55–57, 59, 75–77, 81, 83, 85, 89–90, 92, 94–96, 101–02, 104, 106–08, 110, 112–13, 115, 119, 128–30, 142, 146, 158; necessary 44, 81; trace 59, 90, 96
Nutritional Reform Movement 64
nutritional science 26, 33–36, 70, 77, 87, 93–94, 103, 105, 140
nuts 96, 153

O

obesity 8, 33, 61, 90, 100, 106, 145
omega 3 97, 119
omnivores 68, 87–88
orange flowers 126
organelle 43, 47, 54
organically grown 34, 96–97
osteoporosis 66–67, 100, 115
oxidation 90, 117, 144
oxygen 14, 42, 44, 47, 52, 75, 97, 102, 110, 117–18, 129–30, 138, 145

P

pancreas 93–94, 110, 144
paradigm for human health 5
Parkinson's disease 46
parsley 116
Pasteur, Louis 18
pathogens 9, 15, 17–20, 25, 28, 32, 37–43, 47, 49–51, 53–54, 157–59
Pauling, Linus 131
peach flowers 126
peas: black-eyed 99; pigeon 153
pectin 97
penicillin 18
pepsin 41, 104
pesticides 29, 30
Peyer's patches 128
pH balance 100
phosphorous 115
phytochemicals 47, 55, 59, 83, 85, 96–97, 118, 126, 132, 158

CPSIA information can be obtained at www.ICGtesting.com
Printed in the USA
BVOW05s1538201115

427561BV00004B/11/P

9 780982 290040